TIMOTHY BLOSSOM

OFFICIALLY BRILLIANT

STEVE SLAVIN

MARSHWOOD

Cover created by Matt Maguire—Candescent Press

For children who think differently.

1 TIMOTHY JAMES ARTHUR BLOSSOM

HELLO, I'm Timothy James Arthur Blossom, or Timothy for short. I'm twelve years, three months, five days, and 139 minutes old—or at least I was when I just said it. I've lived at 47 Eaton Drive my entire life. I share the house with my parents and best friend, Schrodinger. He's orange and has only been with us since my last birthday. Before that, my best friend was Albert who had a long green tail and ate worms. But I don't want to say too much about Albert because I've only just recovered from the trauma of watching Dad bury him in the garden next to a tiny cross.

Eaton Drive is in a place called East Winslow, forty miles from London. It's pretty quiet here most of the time, at least it is in *our* street, although the Town Centre's a lot busier than it used to be.

According to Dad, when he was my age, East Winslow was a quaint little village surrounded by farms and woodland. He said the streets were so clean you could practically eat your dinner off the pavement without a plate! Well, I can tell you now, it's definitely *not* something I would've done, even back in the 'good old days.' But I get the point. And that brings me to my next point. People think I'm way too fussy about stuff because I like things to be done in a certain way. But I can't help it; it's just the way I was born. And at twelve years, three months, five days, and 142 minutes old, I guess I'm far too stuck in my ways to change now.

There are lots of other things I'd like you to know about me as well. Let's begin with my favourite place to be in the entire world other than Cornwall and 47 Eaton Drive. I am, of course, referring to the place where only the good dreams come true—AstroWorld, *the store with a universe of galactic gifts.*

I'm not entirely convinced that whoever came up with the strapline, *the store with a universe of galactic gifts,* actually knows the first thing about the multidimensional nature of time and space, but I don't mind too much because AstroWorld is simply such a brilliant place. It doesn't look like much from the outside —just a big grey warehouse in the middle of a car park. But inside, the shelves truly are stacked high with a universe of galactic gifts. The illuminated Earth globe above the main entrance, alone, is enough to pull me closer and closer with its powerful rotating magnetism. I could quite easily spend an afternoon browsing just the telescope section, or with a mug of cocoa in the Stargazer Café, admiring those magnificent hanging models of the Solar System. These, by the way, are currently on special offer at twenty per cent off. A bargain if only I could convince Dad to get his wallet out. Unlikely, I think.

We have a rule that we only visit AstroWorld on Sundays. There's simply not enough time during the week after school, and its cosmic aisles are far too busy on Saturdays. And if there's one thing I hate more than tying shoelaces, Brussels sprouts, and clothes that are too tight, it's crowded places. In fact, if it were down to me, people would be totally banned from all public spaces—especially when *I'm* in them. This would include trains, buses, libraries, pavements, schools, museums, beaches in Cornwall, and the Scottish Highlands—because I would like to visit them one day: in peace.

It may sound strange to people who don't know me, but generally, I like things to be left or right, up or down, right or wrong, black or white, round or square, fast or slow, hot or cold. I really can't stand things that are in-between, like midnight and midday, and soup that's thick enough to be stew.

Here are some more things that I don't like:

- Revolving doors
- Crying babies
- People coming to visit
- School
- Plans changing at the last minute
- Sport
- Secrets
- Parties
- Having friends

I could go on, but I think you get the idea.

Mum said the list of things I don't like is so long it

could reach all the way to the moon. She obviously doesn't have a clue about Einstein's Theory of Relativity—or gravity, for that matter. If she did, she wouldn't make such statements. In any case, she was smiling when she said it. And I read recently on *10 things to know about people.com,* that if a person says something that isn't true, whilst smiling, they are almost certainly telling a joke. And jokes are things that baffle me the most. I mean, words are nothing but sound waves interrupting the air in which they vibrate. What could possibly be funny about that?

Dad tells jokes sometimes, to make me feel less stressed out on train journeys. They usually begin with the words, 'Knock, knock'. And after he's recovered from the embarrassing laughing fit that begins before he's even delivered the punchline, he'll say, 'Why aren't you laughing? Didn't you get it?'

To which I'll reply, 'Get what, exactly?'

Then he'll say, 'THE JOKE TIMOTHY—THE JOKE!'

To which I'll respond, 'Yes, I did, actually, but no one knocks on doors anymore, they use doorbells and social media.'

Then Dad will say, 'Come on, Son, lighten up. Have you had a humour bypass or something?'

I'll inform him that it's not medically possible to have a humour bypass. Then Dad will stop smiling and say, 'Christ, I wish I'd never asked. Never mind, read your book, we'll be there soon!'

Another thing I'd like you to know about me is that I have rules. Lots of rules. Obviously, I can't mention all of them, because that would take too long. But here are a few examples:

- Lunch: first I eat the greens, then the potatoes, and then the carrots. Each item of food must be separated by at least two centimetres to avoid cross-contamination.
- My bedroom: no one, other than Mum, Dad, and Schrodinger are allowed in there. It's where I keep all of my special stuff, and I wouldn't want any of it to go missing.
- Socks: must be worn inside out so the ridges don't dig into my toes.
- Personal contact: I do not shake hands or give hugs. I do not share seats with strangers on the train or talk to people on the phone.

- Conversation: I must always begin my sentence again from the beginning if I'm interrupted.
- Time: I will not get up in the morning until the numbers on my retro-style LED clock add up to an *even* number. 07:01:34, for example, is okay, because it makes forty-two. Then I must jump out of bed with my eyes closed to avoid seeing the numbers tick over to the next digit.

Like I said before, some people might think I'm strange. But it's just the way I am—the way I've *always* been.

I must admit, though, rules really stress me out. But I get even more stressed out if I try to ignore them. They follow me everywhere and force me to do things I don't want to do. Worse still, I never know when a new one is going to appear. They creep up on me during the night when I'm fast asleep, and for some reason, the next day I will no longer be able to walk on a paving stone if it has a crack in it. Or I'll need to touch the doorknob eight times before I can put my key in the lock.

I wish I could get rid of my rules and be like a 'normal' person who doesn't care about things so much. Sometimes I even wish I could be a bit more like Adrian Wilkes. He sits next to me in class and doesn't seem to care about *anything*. Not unless you include aspiring to be the most annoying person on the entire planet. In my opinion, he hit *that* target the first day I met him.

But I suppose the biggest problem with having so many rules, is remembering the ones *I've* created, and the ones someone else has told me to follow. For example, I wouldn't get in trouble if I ignored the rule that forces me to leave a space between each colouring pencil on my homework desk. But I *would* be in serious trouble if I ignored Mum's rule about not leaving the freezer door open after putting the ice cream back. I wouldn't get in trouble if I forgot to count the cartoon planets on my bedroom wallpaper four times over before going to sleep. But I *would* be in trouble if I didn't stick to Mr Willowby's rule about completing my homework on time. He's my science teacher, by the way. I'll tell you more about him later.

But, anyway, that's enough about rules for now. Even talking about them is stressing me out.

And now for the thing I've been saving till last to tell you, the thing I'm most proud of, the special thing that everyone needs to know about me. It's that I am, without the slightest shadow of a doubt, the brainiest kid in Highcrest Manor School. And quite possibly all of East Winslow. At least when it comes to astronomy in particular, and science in general. It's not an exaggeration to say that I know more about space than anyone I've ever met. Even more than Mr Willowby, who's supposed to be the ultimate expert on these things—not including Einstein, of course.

Dad says that one day I'll probably work for NASA and be the first boy from East Winslow in orbit. 'I can just see the headlines now—' he always jokes. *'Timothy Blossom of 47 Eaton Drive, steers the international space station to the edge of the known universe!'*

'But that's impossible, the universe is too vast. I'd be dead by the time I got there!' I remind him every time he cracks the same stupid *dad* joke. The one that only he finds amusing.

But being so good at astronomy in particular, and science in general does have its drawbacks. My clever thoughts light up the parts of my brain that other people don't appear to have. This leaves all the 'normal' bits that other people *do* appear to have, totally in the dark. I have what's called an uneven skill set. This means I'm totally off-the-scale-brilliant at some things, and totally off-the-scale-hopeless at others. It's just the way I'm wired. It's also the reason Dad keeps saying, 'For God's sake, Timothy, why did you do that? I thought you were supposed to be the brainiest boy in East Winslow!'

Well, I *am* the brainiest boy in East Winslow— just not in a way that makes Dad happy.

2 HIGHCREST MANOR SCHOOL

I CAN REMEMBER my first day at Highcrest Manor School as though it were yesterday. In fact, it could have been yesterday. Nothing much has changed around here since I arrived two years ago. I still share a desk with stupid Adrian Wilkes, and Clare Feathersdale still shares the desk in front of ours with her best friend, Amanda Goldbloom. Mr Willowby is still teaching us stuff about science I knew when I was eight-years-old, and I can still go an entire day staring out of the window at pigeons landing on the fence without saying a single word.

According to some tests I had recently, my vocabulary is actually well above average for my age. But it's also 'limited in scope and reciprocation.' I don't exactly know what this means, but what I *do* know, is that when I get going, I can talk for absolutely ages about Einstein and how the universe began. Mr Willowby says I'm 'quite the mad professor.' I like the 'professor' bit, but I'm not sure how politically correct it is to call someone 'mad' these days. But I guess he doesn't mean any harm.

And as for Mum, well she's always going on about how communication is a two-way thing. She says I need to listen more to what other people are saying. 'Life does not always revolve around *you*, Timothy!' She keeps reminding me. But, quite honestly, I've never been particularly interested in what other people are saying. I've got too many brilliant thoughts of my own to talk about. Life is far too short to waste time listening to other people's pointless drivel.

These days, I hardly even bother putting my hand up in science when Mr Willowby asks one of his pathetic questions...

'Okay class, who can tell me how many planets there are in the solar system?'

I mean, *really*... what's the point, everyone knows the answer to *that* question. Everyone, that is, apart from Adrian Wilkes. He'll put his hand up and say something stupid like, 'There are a hundred and twenty planets in the solar system, Sir, and Mars is made of chocolate.'

Quite frankly, I refuse to be associated with such an embarrassing lizard-wort-turtle-scrank. I'll slide over as far away from him as possible—until my books are balancing on the edge of the table—then use my hand to block any sight of him. But I'll still hear him sniggering away under his foul breath, because he thinks that being annoying is such an incredibly brilliant thing to be.

Once, Adrian put his hand up and said, 'But why are you asking *us*, Sir, don't you know the answer or something? I thought you were supposed to know *everything*.'

Well—everyone in the room gasped and stared at Mr Willowby to see what his reaction was going to be. His reaction was to give Adrian a double detention. One for being rude, and another for being 'An Adrian.'

'Oh my God—that's so unfair!' Adrian moaned under his breath, 'I didn't do anything!'

If it were down to me, I would have given him at least ten detentions for being an Adrian, and another ten for being the most annoying person I've ever met.

But then, I don't make the rules around here, Ellen Ford does. She's the headteacher.

To be honest, I wish I didn't have to share a desk with *anyone*. When I first started at Highcrest, I'd stack my books into a border fence across the centre of the desk. But it didn't stop Adrian peeking over the top to steal my answers. Then I made the wall even higher by balancing my lunchbox and a rolled-up jacket on top. But when Mr Willowby saw what I was up to, he told me to dismantle the structure immediately. He said, 'Walls create barriers to communication.' And I totally agree. That's exactly why I built it in the first place!

According to *10 things to know about people.com,* Adrian and I are 'acquaintances'. This is quite a bit less than being friends, but quite a bit more than not knowing each other from Adam (whoever he is).

Clare and Amanda are friends. They do things like link arms in the playground and take bites out of each other's sandwiches at lunchtime. YUK! They have sleepovers and visit each other's houses after school to study. They call themselves 'homework buddies.' I certainly wouldn't want anyone coming over to *my* house every night after school to study. The thought of being Adrian Wilkes' homework buddy would be like the worst nightmare I've ever had—and trust me, I've had some pretty bad ones.

Still, I suppose it could be worse. I could have been in a class with *Billy Farmer:* that evil, disgusting kid who called me a weirdo when I was seven. I'm not sure I'll EVER get over the trauma of *that!*

3 THE TESTS

WHEN MUM TOLD me I was having a day off school, I was elated. She said I needed to have some special tests at a local clinic to see how clever I was. Finally, a chance to have my unique intellect officially recognised. The government would probably even fix one of those circular blue plaques to the front of our house. It would state in gold lettering:

'Timothy Blossom—the cleverest boy in East Winslow lives here.'

The Gazette would run a story on me and the paparazzi would be all over the place, hiding behind Mum's lavender bush and in the garden shed, harassing me for a picture and a comment every time I left the house. And because of my celebrity status, I might even get my own desk in school. One that I wouldn't have to share with *you know who.*

I must admit though, I was pretty disappointed with the way things turned out. *None* of the tests were about science. Quite frankly, it was all a bit boring. I had to memorise loads of words and numbers, and repeat as many of them back as I could in thirty-seconds. Then I had to arrange coloured shapes so that the pictures lined up. Yawn!

'Excellent!' The testing lady said after each task. Then she'd make lots of notes on her computer. I thought this was probably a good sign and meant there were a ton of good things to say about me. But then she asked a bunch of totally irrelevant questions like, 'Do you like friends coming over to your house?' To which I replied, 'Definitely *not*. Friends serve no purpose whatsoever. They are a complete waste of mine and Schrodinger's time. And that's *all* I have to say on the matter!'

Then she asked, 'Would you rather go to a museum, a library, or a party?'

And I said, 'Do you *really* have to ask?! OBVI-OUSLY, I'd rather go to AstroWorld.'

This made her scrunch her eyebrows together in a sort of confused way, probably because AstroWorld wasn't mentioned on her list of possible answers. She didn't know which one to tick and made a quick squiggly note on the paper instead.

Her final question was, 'Do you enjoy jokes?'

I told her that Dad's jokes were designed to entertain people born no later than 1952. And that words should *only* be used to convey important information about interesting, scientifically proven facts. I sat back in my chair and folded my arms.

Finally, after what felt like a week, but was probably only an hour or so, the testing lady put her pen down, and said, 'Thank you, Timothy. You did *really* well.'

By this, I thought she meant I'd definitely done enough to earn top-spot on her chart of epic braininess, or at least somewhere in the top one per cent of the top one per cent. I thought she'd say something like, 'WOW! You are, without a shadow of a doubt, the cleverest twelve-year-old I've ever met.' She'd hand me a certificate I could stick on my bedroom wall and email my test results to NASA for further analysis. But instead, she led me out into the waiting room, where Mum had been drinking coffee and reading magazine articles on 'how to turn your house into a dream home for under £200.'

'Thank you, Mrs Blossom,' the testing lady said. 'I'll be in touch, just as soon as I have some news.' She smiled at me and disappeared back inside her testing room.

Mum and I were soon scoffing double-veggie-whoppers and French fries at the Burger Palace in the High Street. I was pretty stressed out and tired from all the tests and didn't feel like talking. Just as well really, Mum spent most of the time sending messages to Dad from her new phone. Personally, I think there should be a law against parents using social media. All of that tapping and beeping was driving me crazy. I would have stuck my fingers in my ears if I hadn't needed both hands to manoeuvre the burger into my mouth.

She eventually put the phone down and picked up her coffee. She looked at me and smiled, but even I could tell it wasn't a *happy* smile. I'm pretty sure Mum was still thinking about those tests. And I figured Dad must have been thinking about them as well because he never usually responds to messages when he's at work. I was convinced that something really big was going on. Something big that I wasn't allowed to know about. And if there's one thing I hate more than Monday mornings, it's other people knowing stuff that I do not.

We left the Burger Palace and headed home; past Felicity's Flowers and the Italian Deli by the traffic lights. Neither of us spoke. My thoughts were consumed by just one movie. One soundtrack that played over and over again. It was that final scene outside the testing lady's office when she'd said: 'Thank you, Mrs Blossom. I'll be in touch just as soon as I have some news.'

Some news about *what?* I wondered...

The testing lady's final words to Mum followed me all the way home and into my dreams. That night, they became hundreds of angry wasps trapped and buzzing inside a spiderweb stretched tightly across my face. Then, suddenly, I was calm, drifting on a boat made from coconut shells and bamboo shoots. Mr Willowby—wearing swimming goggles and a doctor's coat—whispered, 'I'll be in touch just as soon as I have some news.' He disappeared below the waves, and then there was darkness.

'BREAKFAST IS ON THE TABLE!'

Mum knocked loudly on my bedroom door, jolting me awake. It was 07:01:27 and time to get up for school. But all I could think about was: *'Thank you, Mrs Blossom, I'll be in touch just as soon as I have some news, just as soon as I have some news, just as soon as I have some news....'*

I remembered how Mum and the testing lady had looked at each other. As though they were transmitting secret messages that only adults could understand. And if there's something I dislike even more than wholemeal bread, it's secrets. Especially when they're ones involving *me*.

According to *how to tell if someone is lying.com,* people use secrets to keep you in the dark—not literally, of course. But sometimes, secrets are covered up by white lies, and are used to protect people from knowing things that might upset them. Just like when I was five and had a cat called *Newton.* Dad said I wouldn't be seeing Newton again because he'd emigrated to Australia for health reasons. I'm pretty sure *this* was an example of a white lie being used to cover up a secret. And once he said he'd never be able to tell me anything private, because I'm too honest, and would not be able to keep a secret—well... *secret.*

Dad likes our 'man-to-man' chats. It's a chance for

him to share some of his hard-earned wisdom. He'll say things like, 'To get on in this world, Son, you have to bend the truth occasionally.' Even though I've made it perfectly clear, at least a thousand times, that words cannot be bent. But if they're said loudly enough in a big room with hard walls, they'll bounce around all over the place in ever-decreasing decibels until they can no longer be heard.

I wish Dad had studied physics at school. Then he'd know what I was talking about and we could have man-to-man chats about stuff that *really* matters.

4 FRANK AND LESLIE

THE WORST THING about parents is when their friends drop by for a visit. All of that embarrassing air-kissing-on-both-cheeks stuff. YUK! Never mind all the hugging and handshaking and pointless small talk. And you know they'll do it all again when it's time to leave. And you wonder why I refuse to have a social life?!

Then, after all the greetings have finished, everyone gets a bit more serious and starts complaining about work and politics and the weather and being overweight. I always feel like saying, 'WELL, LEAVE THE CHOCOLATE CAKE ALONE THEN, AND BUY AN UMBRELLA!'

Anyway, by about 8 pm, I'm usually pretty bored,

so I'll sneak upstairs to hang-out with Schrodinger. He's not one for all that embarrassing air-kissing-on-both-cheeks stuff either. That's why we get on so well. We have so much in common.

Luckily, my parents don't have many friends. It's mainly Frank and Leslie. They've been Mum and Dad's best friends for years, so I'm more or less used to them being in the house. But that doesn't mean I feel entirely comfortable when they turn up and start asking me difficult questions.

Questions like:

'How are you, Timothy?'

And: 'How's school going?'

And: 'How did you get so tall?'

I mean, hasn't anyone around here heard of biology?!

At some point (unless I escape upstairs first), Leslie will say how handsome I've become. She'll pull me into her pink chubby chest for a bear hug and attach her fat sloppy lips to the side of my face like a ghastly red-lipstick-limpet. It's horrible. The stuff of nightmares.

But the last time Frank and Leslie came over for wine and sausage rolls—not long after I had those tests to see how brainy I was—Dad got into a massive argument with Frank. It was pretty scary. At one point, I even thought that someone was going to get punched! I made some notes afterwards, just in case I forgot anything. The day went like this: 07:17 AM, I came down to breakfast just as Dad was getting ready to leave for work. He had just enough time to slurp the last of his tea before racing off to catch the 07:34 am train.

'Don't be home late, Bert.' I heard Mum say. 'Remember—Frank and Leslie are coming over tonight to show us their new holiday pictures.'

'Okay, Love, I've gotta run now, I'll see you later.'

Dad grabbed his sandwiches from the table and slammed the door behind him.

8:01 pm

Mum and I were sitting in the living room waiting for Dad to arrive. We had guests.

I heard a key turn in the front door lock. This was followed by leather-heeled footsteps on a hardwood floor.

'BLIMEY, WHAT A DAY!'

It was Dad returning home from work. He was

late—*very* late. His tired voice groaned through the wall as he hung his coat and kicked off his shoes.

'SORRY ABOUT THE TIME, LOVE,' he bellowed from the hallway. 'There was a bit of trouble at the factory. Alf and Charlie are still there sorting out the computers in time for the night shift. What a *blimmin* nightmare. I told them I had to leave because we had guests coming over to show us their boring holiday photos like they do every—*oops!*'

Dad suddenly appeared in the doorway to a seated audience consisting of me, Mum, Frank and Leslie.

'Evening Frank... Evening Leslie... I er—I didn't know you were here already!'

He screwed up his face like he'd said something *really* bad, hoping no one would notice. For a few seconds, there was total silence. Frank and Leslie just sat there on the couch looking like they may never smile again, and Mum's cheeks turned bright pink. I knew something was wrong because *this* only happens when she's either sad, angry, or drinking mulled wine at the School Christmas party.

Now, I'm not very good at judging these things, but I'm pretty sure Dad had done something called 'putting one's foot in one's mouth.' Not literally, of course. That would be an extremely difficult thing to do without at least thirty-years yoga practice on a mountain in Tibet. Dad has only been abroad once, and that was to Spain where they don't do yoga.

'Anyway!' Said Mum, clearing her throat. 'Frank and Leslie were just saying that we should go on holiday with them in June.'

'YES, BERT!' said Leslie (still not smiling). 'Then Frank and I wouldn't need to show you our next collection of BORING holiday pictures—WOULD WE?!' I'm almost certain that Leslie was being sarcastic. This is a form of communication I can just about get my head around if my brain isn't worn out from doing too much homework. Dad must have picked up on this as well because he said: 'Now, there's no need to be sarcastic, Leslie.'

Then Frank said:

'HOW   DARE   YOU   CALL   MY   WIFE SARCASTIC!'

'But she *is* being sarcastic, Leslie was definitely being sarcastic, and we don't like sarcastic people in this house—do we, Barbara?'

'Leave me out of it, Bert. This has got nothing to do with me. You're the one who came home late and in a bad mood.' Mum folded her arms tightly on top of her apron and looked in the opposite direction to where Dad was standing.

'I'M NOT IN A BAD MOOD!' Dad said, in his *almost* angry voice.

'THEN WHY ARE YOU SHOUTING?' shouted Leslie. 'We didn't come over here to get shouted at—did we Frank?'

'NO! We certainly did not!' Frank confirmed.

'I'M NOT SHOUTING, *OKAY!*' said Dad even louder.

'Yes, you are, Bert. I bet everyone in the street can hear you,' said Mum, who I thought was supposed to be on Dad's side but appeared to be agreeing with Frank and Leslie.

I felt like making the point that, technically speaking, not *everyone* who lives on Eaton Drive would be able to hear Dad shouting. Definitely not the ones at the far end by the shops and the noisy traffic, or the Dixons next door who were in Canada visiting family. There was absolutely no way *they* could hear Dad shouting in Ontario!

Then Mum said: 'Stop acting so childishly, Bert, you're embarrassing yourself.'

But Dad wasn't listening. He looked at Frank and Leslie and said: 'I wish I hadn't come home. I've got better things to do than sit here all night listening to the pair of you waffling on about how you lost your passports in Rome or got delayed at Heathrow due to fog. It's the same thing every single blasted year!'

Then Dad went into this long mocking rant. He began speaking through his nose, pretending to be Frank:

'*Now, here's a picture of Leslie standing by the pool in Torremolinos, and here's one of me on the beach in Skegness. Oh, and you'll like this one, it's Leslie eating vanilla ice cream. If you look really closely, you can just about see the raspberry syrup dripping down her arm. We laughed for hours when that happened. She had wasps chasing her all day long... HA, BLASTED, HA! READ MY LIPS FRANK. READ MY LIPS LESLIE. I DO NOT WANT TO SEE ANY MORE OF YOUR BORING HOLIDAY PICTURES. NOT THIS YEAR. NOT NEXT YEAR. NOT ANY OTHER YEAR! AM I MAKING MYSELF CLEAR?*'

I'd never seen Dad so angry. I didn't realise his voice could be so big and scary. I genuinely thought he might self-combust, leaving slimy brain cells dripping from the ceiling. Or that he might have a heart attack, or punch Frank on the nose and go to jail for ten years. Then Mum would divorce him and I'd get thrown out of school, then Schrodinger would be taken into care and I'd never see him again. The situation was getting seriously out of control, and I didn't like it. Then, for some reason, everyone stopped talking and a strange calmness filled the room. It was the type of silence that comes with a sort of background hiss.

I held my breath with my fingers in my ears for as long as I could, hoping the shouting wouldn't start again, and then the most unexpected thing happened. Dad sat down on the couch next to Frank and put his head in his hands (in a manner of speaking). He had a crack in his voice that meant he was trying not to cry.

'Look... Frank, Leslie, Barbara, I'm sorry, okay. I didn't mean what I said. It's just that things are a bit stressful at work at the moment. It looks like the company will be making some cuts, *restructuring* they're calling it. But what it really means is that the whole team, Charlie, Alf, Bernice and me, will be getting the chop. What will I do? I'll be fifty-three next year. I'll be past it, finished, washed up, a has-been. No one will want to employ an old bloke like me, will they? I'll be lucky to get a job sweeping the streets for a minimum wage. I just don't know what I'm going to do.'

Dad turned to Mum and said: 'Sorry you had to hear it like this, Love. I've known for a while now. I just couldn't quite bring myself to tell you. I didn't want you to worry.'

Then Frank—who was Dad's best friend again—said: 'Don't worry, mate, something will turn up, you'll see.'

'I hope so Frank, I really hope so.'

I hardly slept that night. Most of it was spent tossing and turning in the dark. It was hard to tell what were thoughts and what were bad dreams. It was all just one big mush of sadness.

I'd always thought that being a grown-up would be easy and that being a child was far more complicated. I mean, there was school, homework, trying to *fit-in,* stroppy teachers, annoying classmates, unfair bedtimes, itchy uniforms, exams, boring lessons and being told to go to your room all the time. But now, all I could think about was Dad shouting at Frank and Leslie, and wondering what the consequences would be. Was it normal for grown-ups to be so angry with each other? Would Frank and Leslie ever show us their boring holiday pictures again? Would we have to give the Eiffel Tower fridge magnet present back? Was Dad really for the 'chop' at work? And why do they call losing your job 'getting the chop' anyway? And if Dad really was *finished,* would we have to move out of our house and live in cardboard boxes down by the canal with all the other people who got the chop?

It was clear that being old—nearly fifty-three—like Dad, was every bit as stressful as being nearly thirteen, like me. Suddenly, the future looked a whole lot bleaker.

5   I THINK WE SHOULD TELL TIMOTHY

'I REALLY THINK we should tell Timothy,' I heard Mum say.

I was sitting on the sixth-step down from the top of the staircase. Not only was six an acceptable step to sit on because it was an *even* number; it was also the best step from which to eavesdrop on people speaking in the living room without being seen. Mum was using her serious voice, waving an official-looking letter in Dad's direction. But, he, as usual, was slumped in his armchair; face buried in the acre-wide pages of the East Winslow Gazette.

'Look, Barbara,' he said, 'we discussed this last night. I thought we'd agreed *not* to tell him until he was seventeen. By then he'll be able to cope better with... you know... *things*.'

'NO! YOU said we shouldn't tell him yet—remember?' Mum replied. 'We can't simply ignore this and hope it will all go away. In my opinion, he's old enough to understand. We should tell him as soon as possible, so he's got time to adjust before his exams. The school is bound to know about it by now. What if he finds out, by accident, that he's got—?'

There was a loud creak. I had accidentally stepped on a loose floorboard at the bottom of the staircase, and the noise had made Mum stop mid-flow. She crumpled the mystery letter into a tight ball and stuffed it into the top pocket of her apron.

'We were just discussing how well you were doing at school—weren't we, Bert?' He flicked over to the next page and pretended not to hear.

'But I heard Dad say there was something you shouldn't tell me till I was older. What did he mean? And who was that letter from?' I said, staring at Mum's apron pocket.

'Look, it's really nothing for you to worry about. It's just one of those promotional offers from the bank, that's all.'

Every instinct told me that Mum's explanation had not revealed the entire truth. If that letter really was from the bank, why wasn't it stuck under the palm tree fridge magnet from Miami with all the other letters? Or pinned to the corkboard in the kitchen next to that rubbish picture of a house I drew when I was five?

It was obvious that this line of questioning was not getting me anywhere. So, after Dad said that if he ever caught me eavesdropping from the stairs again he'd ban me from visiting AstroWorld for six weeks, I went back upstairs to my room and spent the rest of the evening lying on my bed. All I could do was shuffle half-heard sentences around in my head and try to connect them to that letter; the one Mum wouldn't allow me to see.

After a while, when my thoughts became too big, I tried to stop them by focusing on my breath. I kept filling and exhaling whilst counting to eight and thinking of a sunny day by a waterfall. This was a tip I'd picked up from *how to stop useless thoughts.com*. But my thoughts were too big for the waterfall. They kept bursting in through the ring of protective white light you're supposed to imagine yourself inside. It was all getting too stressful, so I gave up in the end and decided to call it a night. And what a night it had been!

I climbed into bed and switched the light off. All that remained was the soft orange glow from Schrodinger's tank and the comforting hum of its gurgling oxygen pump.

'Oh well, Schrody, my old and trusted friend, I guess some things we are not meant to know.' He released six large bubbles—code for, 'That's an unusually philosophical approach to take. And, by the way, not so much of the "old" please!' Two cushion-shaped bubbles rose slowly to the surface—code for, 'I hope you sleep well tonight.'

'I hope so Schrody, I really hope so...'

The next thing I knew, I was in a room with grey brick walls. A powerful lamp swung slowly from the ceiling. On each rotation, it focused a powerful blast of blinding white light into my face. Opposite, a sweaty man with a deep voice and a twelve o'clock shadow stared at me. He was from the CIA and had access to important information.

'Tell me what you know,' he kept asking. 'Tell me what you know...'

But I didn't know anything. I tried to run from the room—to find my way back to Eaton Drive, but my legs wouldn't carry me. A loud BANG made my insides jump. And that's when I woke up. It must have been Dad slamming the door as he left for work. Then I heard the dreaded, 'TIME TO GET UP. BREAKFAST IS ON THE TABLE!'

I glanced across at my clock. It was 07:01:03. This was a very, very bad sign. Seven, one and three are all odd numbers, and when you add them together, they *still* come to an odd number. I stared hard at the clock, trying to hold my breath without blinking; until the one became two, and the three became four. But I still couldn't make the numbers *feel* good. I knew I'd not be able to hold my breath long enough for the seven to become eight. So instead, I closed my eyes and prayed the world would explode bigger than the Big Bang. Then I wouldn't ever have to go to school again.

'I CAN'T GO IN TODAY, I DON'T FEEL WELL!' I shouted at Mum who was now standing next to my bed. I pulled the covers over my face—code for, 'I'm definitely *not* going to school today, so don't bother trying to make me.'

I guess she must have got the message, because I didn't see her again till lunchtime when she brought me up a sandwich and tried to get me to discuss how

I felt about 'things'—as she put it. I told her that I think about 'things' all the time. That's the problem. What I *really* wanted was a way NOT to think about 'things' so much. And that I wished I could sleep for a week and wake up without a care in the world.

'I think we all wish we could do that, sometimes,' she said, staring out of the window.

As usual, Mum hadn't come up with any answers that made me feel better. And this is exactly why it's such a waste of time talking about my feelings. There's never a conclusion. Just lots of clever words that sound good at the time. But nothing ever changes. I guess I'll always be Timothy Blossom of 47 Eaton Drive. Officially, the most stressed-out kid in East Winslow.

6 THE DAWN RAID

4:22 am

IT WAS the darkest hour before the dawn, and soon all would be revealed. Schrodinger and I had spent the night going over the plans and now it was time for action.

'Good luck,' he signalled by releasing eight medium-sized bubbles. I gave him the thumbs up and threw the covers back.

Armed with my AstroWorld Space Torch (the type with three switchable colours) I slipped quietly out into the unlit hallway. Guided by the narrow beam of light, I crept carefully along the corridor, past Mum and Dad's room on the right and the bath-room on the left. Only the occasional drop from a leaky tap broke the dawn silence. In front of me, the staircase descended steeply into the darkness.

To avoid the creaky steps, I swung my leg over the shiny wooden handrail and slid to the bottom. I dismounted with nothing more than a friction burn to my inner-thigh and turned to view the path ahead: to the kitchen, where Mum's apron and the scrunched-up mystery letter hung tantalisingly on a hook by the window. Soon, its secrets would be mine.

Carefully, I stepped from the warm hall carpet onto the kitchen floor's cold ceramic tiles. They felt hard and crinkly, yet strangely soothing on my skin; an unexpected massage, temporarily throwing me from my mission. *'Focus, Timothy, focus,'* I kept saying to myself. I pointed my torch towards the coat hooks on the far wall, and there, aglow in the piercing beam of my AstroWorld Space Torch, was Mum's flowery apron. My heart pounded. All I had to do was cross the kitchen floor without bumping into the wine rack, the dustbin, and the cupboard with silver saucepans hanging from it.

Finally, with trembling hands, I reached into the apron's top pocket and removed the crumpled letter. I ironed out the creases with the same hand in which I held my torch. This sent a dancing beam of light bouncing around the ceiling, the walls, and the floor. Then suddenly, I heard footsteps on the stairs. Heavy, grown-up footsteps, thumping closer and closer. I panicked and quickly stuffed the mystery letter back into Mum's apron without even the briefest glimpse of its intriguing contents.

From around the corner, long shadows of feminine fingers reached for the switch on the wall. I heard a CLICK and the room was ablaze with dazzling light. I thrust my hand to my face to shield my eyes from the explosion of white. Between my fingers, I could see Mum. She was standing by the kitchen door wearing a red dressing gown and fluffy pink slippers.

'What on *earth* are you doing down here at this time of the morning?!' She asked in a way that made me wonder if I was in trouble.

'I... I was thirsty and wanted to test out my new torch.' I replied, hoping that I hadn't bent the truth so much it had become a lie. But I suppose I was sort of telling the truth. After all, it had been fun trying out my new torch, and a glass of water *did* suddenly sound like a good idea.

Then Mum said, with one of those smiles she makes when she thinks she knows something you don't want her to know about: 'Are you sure there's not another reason you're down here so early?'

She gestured towards the fridge and said, 'You weren't thinking of taking a slice of grandma's home-made chocolate cake, were you? I've been saving that for Sunday. Frank and Leslie are coming over. They've just got back from Bulgaria.'

I looked down at the floor and nodded. I suppose this was what Dad had meant by 'bending the truth'. It certainly seemed like an easy way of not getting into trouble. Mum smiled. She took the cake from the fridge and cut me a thin slice. 'There you go,' she said. 'But don't let your father know. Once he sees a bit's missing, he'll polish off the rest in one go, and he's bursting out of his shirts as it is!'

I switched off my torch and carried the cake up to my room, scoffing the tasty slice in two big yummy bites, then brushed the crumbs from my chest onto the carpet. I lay on my bed watching the sky lighten through the window and counted the planets on my AstroWorld wallpaper four times over without stopping. I tried to count them another four times, but it had been a long night and I could barely keep my eyes open.

My mission may have failed, but at least my belly was full, and that was enough for now. The debrief with Schrodinger would have to wait till later. All I wanted to do now was sleep.

7 SHOELACES

7:13 am

I KNEW this was going to be a rubbish day. Things began to go wrong from the moment I woke up. Firstly, my red, white and blue Apollo 12 branded toothpaste had gone hard. This meant I had to use the green slimy stuff Mum says is better for my teeth; even if it *does* look like a disgusting sloppy slug on a brush. It reminds me of something Bear Grylls would eat in the Australian outback.

And then things got even worse when I couldn't find my new school bag. I had to use the old one that was covered in at least a centimetre of dust. Then I got upset because everything was going so wrong and called Mum an evil old woman because they were the best angry words I could think of.

My exact words were: 'I'M NOT GOING TO SCHOOL TODAY, YOU EVIL OLD WOMAN!'

Then, when I finally got to school, the first thing I heard was: 'Oy, brainbox, why do you always wear those stupid slip-on Velcro shoes?!'

I looked down at my shoes and said: 'BECAUSE I DO—OKAY?'

Adrian laughed, and said: 'But why? Don't you know how to tie your shoelaces or something?'

Then I said: 'SHUT UP ADRIAN, JUST SHUT UP, OR I'LL—'

Luckily, I didn't have to come up with a punishment plan for Adrian because Mr Willowby lost his temper and shouted: 'OKAY BOYS, NO ARGUING IN CLASS, *SOME* PEOPLE ARE TRYING TO CONCENTRATE ON THEIR WORK!'

The truth is, I wear slip-on shoes with Velcro straps because—and I'm really embarrassed to admit this, but Adrian was right—I really *don't* know how to tie my own shoelaces. I can't open a bag of crisps or do the buttons up on my school shirt either. My fingers are simply not built for doing such fiddly tasks.

When I first started at Highcrest, Mum told the lady in Student Services about my 'shoelace problem.' She said I could wear shoes without laces instead. So, Mum bought me these ugly black things with Velcro straps that make me feel sad, stupid and useless. And now, I'm officially the only kid in Highcrest who wears such monstrosities on their feet. In fact, I'm surprised Adrian Wilkes hasn't made fun of my slip-on shoes before. Probably, because he's such a slow, slug-worm-dungbat, he simply hasn't noticed —even though I've sat next to him every single day for two years. Apart, that is, from Saturdays, Sundays, bank holidays, teacher-training days, diversity days, trips to Cornwall with Mum and Dad days, and Christmas days.

But today—the day I knew would be the worst day *EVER* from the moment I woke up—was the day I realised that I was even more different to everyone else at Highcrest than I'd previously thought. I mean, why *can't* I tie my own shoelaces? Even that wombat-weasel-skunk Wilkes can tie his. Not that it's particularly obvious. They never stay done up for long. They're usually dragging along through the playground puddles until a teacher shouts, 'Oy, Wilkes, do your laces up before someone trips over them!'

And this reminds me of the rule I've not mentioned yet: the rule about never taking my shoes off in a public place. The straps make this terrible crackling sound when I pull them apart. They're like the world's loudest firecrackers. And trust me, it's definitely *not* a good idea to draw any unnecessary attention to yourself in school. You know how cruel kids can be.

Mum says that Adrian only does things to make me angry because he's jealous. Jealous because I've got my own brilliantly special way of doing things. But I'm not convinced she really thinks this. What she probably means, but doesn't want to say, is that Adrian makes fun of me because he thinks I'm strange. I guess she's just trying to help me feel better about myself. And quite honestly, when it comes to feeling better about myself, I need all the help I can get.

'Don't worry Timmy, you'll get the hang of it one day,' Mum says, whenever I can't do something even a five-year-old would find easy. But the truth of the matter is I'm just as useless at looking after myself at twelve years, five months, and twenty-six days of age, as I ever was. I'm destined to remain a big useless baby till the day I die. A big useless baby who needs their mother to get them dressed each morning. To spread butter on their toast and thread their belt through the loops to stop their trousers falling down.

Sometimes I wish I didn't have to be so brainy and have such brilliantly special ways of doing things. Sometimes I just want to be average; normal, like everyone else.

Adrian Wilkes was right. I really am just a big hopeless baby who can't even tie his own shoelaces. How pathetic is that? How pathetic am I?

8 ME VERSUS THE INTERNET

HOWEVER HARD I TRIED, I could not stop thinking about that secret letter. Or, for that matter, the conversation between Mum and Dad in the living room a few days earlier. Somehow, I needed to find out what was going on. So, the following Saturday, I decided to spend the entire day investigating at my computer.

First, I searched the internet for information on how to hire a private detective, and how to become a spy. Then I typed 'how to tell if your parents are lying' and 'ten ways to tell if your child is brainy.' Okay, so this last one wasn't totally relevant, but it's easy to get side-tracked on the internet. In a flash, there were adverts all over the page for lie detector kits and articles on how to translate body language into words even I can understand. This was all useful stuff, but not exactly what I was looking for.

Then, by accident, I clicked on an advert for organic dog food. This appeared because the previous day I'd searched for, 'how to stop the neighbours' dog barking every time you walk past?'

I am, of course, referring to the wild beast commonly known as *Trevor*—the golden retriever who lives next door.

'Buy some noise-cancelling headphones...' Seemed to be the most useful piece of advice on offer. So I clicked, and was immediately bombarded with pictures of death-metal rock musicians and construction workers wearing ear protection. So I typed, 'how can I stop adverts about headphones appearing on my computer?' Instantly, my screen was splattered with special offers on cybersecurity software. I ended up scrolling through pages and pages of articles on how *not* to get hacked by people in countries I'd never even heard of.

I was getting nowhere and even Schrodinger was losing interest. He'd stopped blowing bubbles and was descending slowly to the gravelly bottom of his tank. Behind him was a dark brown trail.

'Urrgg, Schrodinger, that's disgusting!' I said loudly in my thought voice. He replied with a great big single bubble that rose and popped on the surface —code for, 'Oops, sorry you had to see that!' He flicked his tail and vanished into a swirl of murky water. It was like Schrodinger had read my mind. So I typed into the search bar: 'Does my goldfish *really* know what I'm thinking?'

There weren't many relevant results for this, only about a million or so. But just as I was ready to give up, halfway down on page sixty-four, I saw an online course entitled: *Remote Viewing—A Beginner's Guide* by ex-CIA agent Robert J. Hoffenbaker.

According to Robert J. Hoffenbaker, the KGB had trained some of their agents to spy on American military bases using only the power of thought. A skilled remote viewer, as they were called, could, apparently, sit safely in their Moscow office and visualise top-secret technology being developed at a place called Area 51, deep in the Nevada desert. The Americans also had a team of remote viewers. They'd been spying on the Russians for decades.

This got me thinking. Just imagine how great it would be if I could travel anywhere in the world using only the power of thought. I'd never have to leave the house again! No more noisy train stations where people bump into you and never say sorry. Or people bashing their suitcase into yours at the airport as if your suitcase had a great big sign on it saying:

'FEEL FREE TO BASH INTO ME. DON'T WORRY, THERE'S NOTHING OF ANY GREAT VALUE INSIDE. ONLY MY LAPTOP, MY BOOKS ON ASTRONOMY, MY BRAND NEW ELECTRIC TOOTHBRUSH THAT SPINS AT 3000 REVOLU-TIONS PER SECOND. AND MY STUFFED BEAR —*HAROLD*—THAT I'VE HAD SINCE I WAS TWO YEARS OF AGE. BUT DON'T TELL ADRIAN WILKES BECAUSE HE'LL THINK I'M A BABY!'

Anyway, getting back to the subject of remote viewing, I began to wonder if I could use the tech-nique to eavesdrop from my bedroom on Mum and Dad, the next time they have one of their secret conversations. Even Schrodinger appeared excited by my breakthrough. He released sixteen enormous bubbles—code for, 'You should *definitely* sign up for Robert J. Hoffenbaker's remote viewing course.'

But after some quick calculations, I realised that even with the fifteen per cent discount on offer, the cost of the course would add up to more than eleven years' worth of pocket money. So I typed, 'how to learn remote viewing without paying.' I waited, and waited, and waited some more, as my computer trawled the greatest reservoir of knowledge ever to have existed. And then, finally, some really good news and some really bad news—24,000,760, 376 results in 2.1 seconds! It actually felt more like 2.1 *minutes*, but then, the WI-FI in East Winslow can be a bit slow on Saturdays when all the kids are at home playing pointless games on their computers. This was obviously going to take longer to research than I'd thought.

Then because I'd typed in, 'how to do remote viewing without paying,' there were suddenly thousands of articles about 'how to grow rich while you sleep.' And 'ten free ways to unlock your true destiny and marry the person of your dreams.' YUK!

It was all getting too much. 'NO!' I screamed at the internet. 'STOP DOING THIS. LEAVE ME ALONE!'

My head began to swim, not literally of course, because I don't like swimming pools. They smell of chlorine—a variety of which was used to poison soldiers in World War 1. And I certainly wouldn't want anything like that happening to me. Exhausted, I turned the computer off and lay on my bed, wondering why the World Wide Web was so annoying.

After my head had cleared a bit, it occurred to me that you have to tell the internet *exactly* what you mean. If you do not, all manner of unexpected things would result. Just like in real life. Like when Mum once said: *'Quick,* Timothy, get your skates on, you're going to be late for school!'

So I did—I literally put my skates on and caught my wheels on the carpet. I bumped down the stairs and whacked my head on the bannister.

Mum said: 'NO TIMOTHY, I didn't actually mean *put your skates on!* I meant—oh… never mind!'

But by then I was lying spread-eagled and upside down with my wheels spinning in different directions. I won't be misinterpreting *that* request anytime soon.

Apparently, I'd gotten hold of the *wrong end of the stick*, again. It took me a while to understand what Mum meant by this. Whenever she says it, I still get pictures in my head of rabid *Trevor the Retriever* from next door chewing on a soggy saliva stick. YUK!

Anyway, it was now late afternoon, and all of that internet surfing had turned my brain into a dull, foggy mush. I closed my eyes, and the next thing I knew I was floating, ghost-like, along the hallway, down the stairs and into the kitchen. Everything was black and white with a hint of green, as if viewed through a pair of those night-vision glasses soldiers wear in the desert. I shone my torch to inspect the aprons hanging on the wall by the sink, but its light was eaten by the room's unnatural darkness. I was terrified, but I could not run. I could not speak, and I could not hear Mum's slow-motion words fall from the mouth that was no longer hers.

With a JOLT, I was back in my room, drowsy but awake. I couldn't work out if it was morning and time to get up for school, or evening and time to go downstairs for dinner.

'Wow, Schrodinger, that was the worst nightmare ever.'

He released four different-sized bubbles—code for, 'I know what you mean, once I dreamed I was being chased by a piranha!' And I knew exactly what *he* meant. I also feel like I'm being chased by piranhas: thought-piranhas. They're brown with rows of gnashing teeth. They swim around in my brain eating up all the happiness.

Schrodinger sunk again to the bottom of his tank and disappeared inside a thick clump of seaweed. It had been a long day and I guess he wanted to be alone for a while, to think about stuff without being looked at. Exactly how I feel most of the time. Sometimes I can't believe how similar we are—me and Schrody. The only friend I'll ever need.

9 THE CODE RED

Monday Morning

IT WAS one of those mornings when I couldn't believe how cruel life was for making the day a school day. My belly throbbed red and raw inside like a volcano trying to explode. But it wasn't the type of pain you get when you catch a virus. Or the type of pain that comes from eating infected chicken at a barbecue. It was the pain I get whenever I'm worried about something new happening at school, or before a visit to the dentist. Or when I wake up and realise it's the first day of August. Because August is an in-between month that confuses me. The first bit still feels like summer and people look happy. The men wear thin shirts and the women wear dresses that stop at their knees. And then, for some reason, the head-controller from the government's official weather-control department turns down the heat, and all we'll have to look forward to are months and months of winter gloom.

Mum says that if I stopped worrying about everything so much my belly aches would simply disappear, 'Like a bad dream in the cold light of day,' she'll say when she's in one of her Shakespearian moods. But that's impossible, there are millions and millions and millions of things to be worried about, and not nearly enough daylight in the universe to make them all go away.

My worries are like zombies in a disaster movie. I could chop every single disgusting one into a gazillion tiny pieces, set each piece on fire, then blast all the bits into the unknowable clutches of a faraway black hole, and *still* another thousand thought-zombies would appear from the shadows to haunt me.

I lay beneath the covers for a few more minutes, wondering about the most effective way to kill a zombie. But then I realised what the time was, and if I didn't get up soon, Mum would start knocking on my door again. And if there's anything I hate more than tight, itchy trousers, it's loud banging on my bedroom door.

Somehow, I managed to crawl out of bed, clutching my belly and being extra careful not to wake Schrodinger. He's not generally a morning type of fish, and by the looks of things he'd had quite a night. Seaweed was strewn across his stone arch, and the coloured gravel on the bottom had been whipped into a hill high enough for a prawn to ski down. I was curious to know what had happened, but figured he'd tell me all about it after school.

Mum was right when she'd said that being out in the fresh air would make my stomach ache go away. By the time I got to school, most of the pain had gone. Unfortunately, this did not include the biggest pain of all...

'Oy, brainbox—wanna see my bruise? I fell off my bike on the way to school this morning!' Adrian thrust a grazed left knee onto the desk, knocking my pencil case onto the floor.

'NO, I DO *NOT*—THANK YOU VERY MUCH!

I've got *much* more important things to think about,' I replied, reaching down to retrieve my AstroWorld branded notepad and pens.

'And I think I've broken my elbow as well. Look... it's all wobbly,' he continued, smiling.

'Well, it doesn't look wobbly to *me*. And anyway, if your elbow really was broken, you'd be screaming out in pain, and you are definitely *not* screaming out in pain.'

'AHHH!' He screamed quietly under his breath, so as not to alert Mr Willowby.

Amanda—who Adrian spends *lots* of time trying to impress with his stupid pranks, turned around and glared at him. 'Shut up, you idiot!' She said, in a quiet growl. Her eyes went really wide like they were about to pop out of her head. 'Stop being such a... such a—'

It was like she couldn't think of a bad enough word to say, so made a 'GRRR' sound instead. Clare put a comforting arm around her and whispered, 'Just ignore him, and he'll go away.'

But he didn't, and aimed a scrunched-up piece of paper at their desk and giggled. 'But I really have broken my elbow. Look, it's wobbling all over the place!'

Mr Willowby, who was busy preparing the lesson

from behind his desk, paused and bellowed: 'LOOK! IF YOU DON'T STOP WITH ALL OF THIS NONSENSE ABOUT WOBBLY ELBOWS—YOU'LL GET ANOTHER DETENTION. DO I MAKE MYSELF CLEAR?!'

Adrian immediately stopped being annoying and didn't say a single word for the rest of the morning. A small mercy, when I had so many other much more important things to worry about.

Tuesday Morning

I have decided.

Today, I shall not speak to anyone belonging to the species commonly known as human. This, by good fortune, rules out my one and only true friend, Schrodinger—because he's a fish.

I shall not speak to Dad because he wants me to be a 'normal' boy who likes to play football in the park on Sundays with all the other 'normal' boys. I shall not speak to Adrian Wilkes because that poor excuse for a single-celled amoeba laughed at my Velcro slip-on shoes the other day. I shall not speak to Mr Willowby either, because he recently looked at me in a bad way; just because I reminded him that Pluto is a dwarf planet. It is definitely *not* a real planet like Mars or Venus as he'd so foolishly stated in class. I said that if he was anything resembling a *good* teacher, he'd know this and would not make such elementary mistakes!

Neither shall I speak to Clare Feathersdale or Amanda Goldbloom. Not that I've ever spoken to either of them before, or them to me. But if for some reason, they *did* start talking to me today, I would absolutely definitely ignore them, anyway, just to make the point that I was in a really... *really* bad mood.

Today, I shall not say 'Thank you' to the old lady who stands by the side of the road with a stop sign to make sure kids cross safely. And I shall not even speak to Mum when I get home after school. Not because she's done anything wrong. I just want her to know how utterly, devastatingly, life-changingly upset I've been since I woke up this morning. I don't remember exactly what it was that had been bothering me, but it must have been something pretty terrible. Bad enough for me to initiate a *code-red*. This is defined in the dictionary of special words I'm currently compiling, as:

The state of verbal shut down I enter when overcome by especially worrying circumstances.

During a code-red, I become a nuclear submarine on high alert. I batten down the hatches and *dive, dive, dive* to the bottom of the deepest thought-ocean. There, I remain for exactly twenty-four hours, and not a second less.

One more important thing I should say about a code-red, is that if I'm forced to communicate before its time has elapsed, it must begin again for another twenty-four hours. Once, I went an entire week without speaking. By the Sunday evening, my words had disappeared so far off into space I never thought I'd hear them again. I ended up at the hospital with doctors looking down my throat, and in my ears, and up my nose—because, *obviously*, that's where my words had disappeared to!

They checked my height and weight and strapped a blow-up rubber band around my arm to test my blood pressure. Then they took magnetic pictures of my brain. They put me in a noisy, white tube just wide enough to breathe in and told me not to move for thirty-seconds. But still the doctors couldn't work out where my words had gone. Just think how much time and expense could have been saved if only they'd asked me about my code-red—not that I would have told them, of course.

Mum can usually tell when I'm in a code-red. She knows it means I'm upset about something that cannot be discussed until I resurface the following morning and activate a *code-green*. This is defined in my dictionary of special words as:

A state of reconnection—emergence from a code-red.

That's when we talk about deep stuff that can only be talked about if I'm drinking hot milk with chocolate sprinkles from my AstroWorld space mug.

'Good morning,' Mum said when I came down to breakfast this morning—before she realised I wasn't speaking to anyone.

'Good morning,' said Dad who was late for work and didn't bother hanging around for the reply I wasn't going to give him anyway.

'Good morning,' Mr Willowby said as I walked into class. I usually ignore him anyway, but today I made extra sure to let him know I wasn't speaking, by looking in exactly the opposite direction. I think he got the message.

'Morning, Brainbox,' Adrian Wilkes mumbled through sneaky bites of a chocolate bar he'd smuggled into class. And still, I remained silent; determined not to violate my code-red.

My day of not speaking to anyone was going nicely to plan. Lunch came and went without speaking, as did afternoon lessons and afternoon break. My walk home from school was also pleasantly communication-free, as was my non-greeting to Mum at the front door when I completely ignored her and ran up to my room.

The evening meal passed without even a hint of a word, and at precisely 9:01 pm, which fortunately comes to an even *ten* when added together, I jumped into bed, happy that, by morning, my words would reappear and I'd allow them to be used again. Unless, of course, we were burgled during the night and I'd have to give a description of the thieves to the police.

I switched off the light and snuggled down under the covers.

'Goodnight,' I transmitted in the direction of Schrodinger's glowing tank. He flipped over and gulped twice—code for, 'And a very good, silent night to you too, Timothy Blossom!'

10 THE SURPRISING THING ABOUT SURPRISES

I'M DEFINITELY NOT a big fan of surprises. Because, when a surprise happens, it means an event is suddenly taking place that I have no control over.

In my opinion, the worst surprises of all are the noisy ones. And at the very top of my list of most-hated-noisy-surprises are balloons that pop unexpectedly. By the time I've closed my eyes and put my fingers in my ears, it's always too late—BANG!

Even the threat of a balloon popping nearby throws my thoughts around like a brain in a tumble dryer. Then, just as I'm recovering from the shock, some stupid kid will pop another one and explode my insides all over again.

But there are lots of other noises I hate as well:

ones I *do* expect to happen. Like when Trevor the Golden Retriever tries to scare me when I walk past.

Trevor doesn't really do much other than bark. And sometimes he can't even be bothered to do that, especially when it's a hot summer's day. He'll just lay there under the hedge pretending to be asleep with one eye open. He's like the world's laziest guard dog until he hears me tiptoeing past. Then, if he's in a bad mood, he'll spring into action, snarling and jumping against the gate like a rabid devil dog with razor-sharp teeth bubbling with saliva.

In my opinion, Trevor has the loudest bark of any dog in East Winslow. But Mum says I shouldn't be frightened because he's never actually bitten anyone. And that his bark is almost certainly a million times worse than his bite. She says that Trevor is just being a dog, and all that noise is simply his way of saying hello. If you ask me, it's just Trevor's way of saying, 'I'd like to rip the flesh from your bones and eat you alive—*slowly!*'

But it's not only dogs and balloons that get me stressed out. I have a long list of noises I hate. A very long list, in fact. One that seems to grow longer by the hour. It's pinned to the corkboard organiser hanging on the back of my bedroom door. Whenever I hear a new noise that makes me put my fingers in my ears, I rush home and add it on with a red marker pen.

Among the other noises on my noise-hate-list are: police sirens, ambulance sirens, fire engine sirens, motorbikes, and those annoying moped things that pizza delivery drivers buzz around on—the ones that sound like gigantic angry wasps. I also hate police helicopters that hover over nearby crime scenes for ages looking for criminals. And I hate drunk people who sing in the street on their way home from the pub at night when I'm trying to sleep. I hate people speaking on their phones on the bus, especially when you can hear the other person's tinny voice on the other end. And I hate cars that pull up alongside ours at the traffic lights with loud banging music that makes my insides vibrate.

I also hate mothers with crying babies who sit near me in the café when I'm trying to eat my burger in peace. And I hate that high-pitched beeping noise lorries make when they're reversing to warn people behind.

Other noises I hate are car alarms, smoke alarms, house alarms, and even my own retro-style digital alarm clock with green flashing numbers. At exactly 7 am, the morning after it arrived in the post, it went off like a rocket-bomb-hurricane-volcano-fighter-jet landing in my bedroom. Since then, I haven't used its alarm function once.

The other type of surprise I hate is when there's an unexpected change to the schedule. This means I have to readjust my thoughts, and for some reason, I can't seem to do this very easily.

What confuses me even more is when a change happens to the schedule that I'm convinced will end in disaster, but then the day turns out better than it would have done if everything had gone to plan. Like the time Dad was going to take me to the Apollo exhibition at AstroWorld; something I'd been looking forward to for months. It was a chance for me to experience the wonders of the cosmos without the actual danger of blasting into space above a million gallons of burning jet fuel. But just as we were getting ready to leave for the train station, Dad experienced some unexpected projectile dysfunctions of his own.

We'd just finished scoffing one of Mum's legendary Sunday roasts, when Dad—being Dad— decided to polish off the leftovers from the previous night's Chinese takeaway.

'Waste not, want not,' he kept reminding us as he

shoveled sweet and sour prawns into his mouth with a silver dessert spoon.

Gradually, his face turned a yellow shade of green. He leapt from his seat and ran full-speed up the stairs to the bathroom, slamming and bolting the door behind him. The whole house shook.

'URRGG... URRGG... OH GOD... URRGG... OH NO, NOT AGAIN... URRGG!' Was all that Mum and I could hear through the door as Dad emptied his stomach into the toilet bowl.

'ARE YOU ALRIGHT IN THERE, BERT!' Mum kept calling out.

'Er, yes, Barbara, I'll be fine in a—OH GOD, NO... URRGG... IT'S PROBABLY JUST SOME-THING I... URRGG... ATE... URRGG...!' Dad replied back through the locked door whilst gasping for air.

Mum shook her head in disbelief at Dad's unnec-essary predicament and straightened the picture frames that had wobbled in the hallway.

'Well, it looks like the trip to AstroWorld's off!' She said. 'Never mind, I'll take you to the park instead —sorry, Timmy.'

Now, I've never actually told Mum this, but I hate it when she calls me Timmy. It's a word that nearly rhymes with *Billy*, that stupid boy from school who called me a weirdo when I was seven.

And that reminds me of another incredibly important thing you need to know about me. Once a thought gets stuck inside my head—especially if it's a bad one—it's likely to stay there for a very, *very* long time.

Being called 'Timmy' *and* finding out we were going to the park instead of AstroWorld, were sure signs that the afternoon was going to be a disaster, which it sort of was. But then it turned into something sort of good, but still quite bad—kind of.

I'd been on the swings for around ten minutes when I heard: 'OY, BRAINBOX, WHAT ARE YOU DOING HERE?!'

It was Adrian Wilkes, whose sole purpose in life was still, quite obviously, to be as annoying as humanly possible. Not only in school, but everywhere else in the universe as well.

'Well, if you *must* know, I'm here because my dad was supposed to take me to the Apollo exhibition at AstroWorld, but he threw prawns up all over the bathroom at lunchtime so Mum brought me here instead.'

'AstroWorld? What's *that*?' Adrian asked. 'It

sounds really boring. Like school or homework...'

He stood there for a second or two, scratching his head to warm a brain cell, and said: 'Anyway, why are you here with your mum? Can't you even go to the park by yourself? What a baby!'

He was sort of laughing at me without actually laughing. An angry feeling came over me that was similar to the time a vandal sprayed red, swirly patterns on Dad's garage door.

I suddenly felt brave, like I might lose control of my emotions and punch Adrian really hard. But I'd never actually stood up for myself before, so this was uncharted territory. I had no idea what the consequences would be if I challenged Adrian to a fight.

'SHUT UP, ADRIAN!' I shouted. 'I'M NOT A BABY. And anyway, how come you've never heard of AstroWorld? Doesn't your dad ever take you there?'

By now, my bravery had completely disappeared, as though it had never existed in the first place, and I was worried that Adrian may become angry and resort to violence. But instead, he just carried on swinging, staring blankly into space as if thinking really hard about what I'd said.

He began to swing higher and higher until his seat became level with the bar to which its chains were attached. At one point, I thought he might even go over the top and fly off into the bushes. But gradually, his swing slowed until it matched mine. I must admit, I was pretty relieved to see he wasn't angry, that he wasn't thinking of punching me on the nose. This made me feel brave again.

In the background, I could see Mum sitting on the bench at the far end of the playground. She smiled and waved at me, but I didn't wave back because I quite liked feeling brave and didn't want Adrian to call me a baby again.

After a few minutes' awkward silence, Adrian said: 'I come here on Sundays by myself because I don't exactly have a dad to take me places. Well, I sort of do—have a dad, that is—but I don't see him much. It's complicated. He doesn't live with me and Mum anymore. He's got a girlfriend called Sally. They live in Sussex with my stepsister Rosie and Rosie's stepbrother Ian, who happened because Sally once had a boyfriend called Brendan who worked in the pub where my dad met Sally—or something like that.'

My brain was so busy unravelling the complexities of Adrian's domestic arrangements that I hadn't noticed my swing was barely moving. Adrian leapt from *his* and said, 'Come on, I'll give you a push.'

But before I could say, 'NO DON'T,' because I hate being touched by anyone other than Mum, I could feel the palms of his hands firmly on my back propelling me forward in my seat.

'NOT TOO HIGH, ADRIAN! I DON'T LIKE HEIGHTS, I MIGHT THROW UP!' I shouted—scared I could lose my grip and crash headfirst onto the concrete floor.

'DON'T WORRY, YOU WON'T FALL OFF. TRUST ME, I GO *MUCH* HIGHER THAN THIS. JUST HOLD ON TIGHT AND YOU'LL BE FINE!'

Adrian pushed me higher and higher until all I could see were quick flashes of blue sky and clouds mixed with fleeting glimpses of rapidly approaching ground. Up and down, back and forth I travelled until I was no longer scared. I closed my eyes and threw my head back. I'd never felt so free. I was flying and swooping and soaring again into space; far beyond every fear I'd ever known until I heard Adrian's voice from somewhere miles below.

'Ouch, my arms are aching,' he groaned, and began using his hands like a brake to slow me down. 'There you go. I told you, you'd be safe if you held on tightly and trusted me.'

'TIME TO GO NOW, TIMMY!' Mum's voice

echoed loudly from the bench and across the play area. This was *seriously* embarrassing. All the kids turned their heads to see who 'Timmy' was. They were all younger than me, and none of them were there with their mothers. I pretended not to hear her at first, but to avoid any further announcements, I jumped from the swing and followed her out of the park, ten steps behind, hoping she wouldn't stop to acknowledge me.

'GOODBYE, TIMOTHY BLOSSOM. SEE YOU AT SCHOOL TOMORROW!' I heard Adrian shout as we turned the corner into Ellsworth Lane.

'Goodbye,' I replied in my thought voice—not caring whether he received the message or not.

'Well, that was a pleasant surprise—bumping into your friend, Adrian, in the park, wasn't it?' Mum said when we got home.

'He's *not* my friend, and I didn't bump into him. He's just someone I sit next to in school. I've told you a thousand times, I do not want friends. They're annoying, and you have to speak to them all the time, and invite them over for sleepovers, and buy them

Christmas presents and birthday presents, and play football with them in the park, and message them on Instagram, and sit next to them at lunch. And if your friend is a girl, people say, *"Urrgg, who's going out with Amanda Goldbloom then?"* Or Clare Feathersdale, or even Shelly Evans who everyone says has *lots* of friends who are boys. I just want everything to stay how it is. Just you, me, Dad and Schrodinger.'

I slumped heavily onto the couch and buried my head in a cushion to calm myself down. Through the slowly settling sediment, amongst the weeds of my many tangled thoughts, I began to realise that something big had changed that afternoon. So big that I was faced by questions I'd never worried about before. Such as, is there a scientifically proven method for calculating the exact point at which an acquaintance becomes a friend? And equally, is there a way of knowing the precise moment that someone stops being one? And what if Adrian Wilkes thinks I'm *his* friend, but I don't think he's mine? Won't this just add to the confusion? And what if he doesn't get on with Schrodinger? How awkward would *that* be...?

'Oh well,' I thought, sighing and wishing I was a goldfish. I guess there never will be enough answers for all of life's impossible questions.

11 ADRIAN'S NEW LEAF

SOMETHING REALLY STRANGE had happened to Adrian.

At school—the morning after seeing him in the park—he was like a completely different person. And it wasn't just because he was wearing a bow tie and had brushed his hair. No, it was something much bigger than that. As though he'd had a personality transplant from someone who was at least a million times nicer. Someone far less annoying. Someone infinitely more civilised than the usual Adrian Wilkes.

'Hi Timothy, how's it going?' He asked.

How's *what* going? I wondered.

This was all too confusing. For a start, he'd never

actually called me by my real name before—apart from a couple of times in the park the previous day. Until then I wasn't even sure if he knew what my real name was. Once, for a joke—at least I think it was a joke—he'd even asked if my birth certificate had 'Brainbox' written on it. Pretty dumb really, considering *he* was the one who came up with the stupid nickname in the first place. And I don't remember him being there when my parents had me registered.

Anyway, by 9:30 am, the new Adrian had already beaten his old, *being friendly in class,* record by almost seven minutes. Not bad, considering his previous record was only fifteen-seconds. I must admit, I was impressed. He even smelled different. Sort of clean. Like he'd used soap or something. But I still didn't want him leaning all over me, reading my notes with that hot skunk-breath of his hitting the back of my hand. YUK!

But I wasn't the only one who was confused by the new-improved Adrian. Even Clare and Amanda kept turning around to stare. They had expressions on their faces that I think meant, 'Wow—that's strange!'

I even began to wonder if the old Adrian had a

secret twin, identical in every way but with better personal hygiene.

'Good morning, Clare... Amanda. How are you both this fine day?' He asked—as if quoting directly from *how to be a nice person for beginners.com.*

Clare and Amanda giggled quietly and linked arms.

Mr Willowby was running late that morning and had told everyone to sit quietly whilst he organised things for the first lesson. But this did not prevent Adrian from enquiring into the state of his health.

'Good morning, Sir—how's your day been so far?'

'I'm good, thank you, Adrian. And why are *you* so happy today? Have you won the lottery?'

'No Sir, I've turned over a new leaf. The old me is nothing but a dark and distant memory.'

Well, everyone in the room practically fell off their chairs, howling with laughter. Amanda's face turned bright red. Streams of happy tears poured down her cheeks and onto the floor. Meanwhile, Clare gasped desperately for air, I think she was trying to say, 'OH MY GOD, WHAT THE—!'

For a minute, I thought she was going to pass out, but then she started breathing again and screamed so loudly my eardrums almost burst. Her happy tears fell next to Amanda's and formed a tiny pond of joy.

I suppose I could have tried harder to understand why everyone had found Adrian's comment about 'turning over a new leaf' so hilarious, but I was far more interested in contemplating the exact type of leaf he was referring to. Perhaps something evergreen from a rhododendron bush? Or something gold and crisp from the oak tree in the playground? After all, autumn *was* just around the corner (in a manner of speaking).

I glanced over at Adrian who I figured was also thinking deeply about leaves because his face was as straight as Mr Willowby's. He wasn't laughing either and had totally lost control of the class. He kept shouting, 'BE QUIET!' But no one was listening. Kids were throwing stuff all over the place: pencil cases, rolled-up balls of paper, lunch boxes, items of High-crest branded uniform. It was chaos, and I was worried that something heavy, like a staple gun, may fly across the room and hit me on the head, so I shielded my face just in case.

Suddenly, Mr Willowby let out a deafening: 'QUIET, OR YOU'RE ALL GETTING DETENTION!' I'd never heard anyone shout so loud. I could have sworn the glass shook in the window frames. I half expected him to turn green and ugly and bust out of his shirt.

Gradually, the class became quiet, and everyone, apart from Adrian, returned to normal.

I was used to feeling like the odd one out—the only one who didn't get the joke; who couldn't see the funny side—but I don't think Adrian was. He looked like he was going to cry or something. Like he wished he could have been anywhere else on the planet at that precise moment; just how I feel when I'm sad and embarrassed. I couldn't say for certain, but I'm pretty sure I was experiencing what *psychology for twelve-year-olds.com* calls 'empathy.' Defined as:

The ability to understand the feelings of another person.

Wow! I thought. I never knew I could do *that!*

Anyway, the 'new' Adrian was pretty quiet for the rest of the day. He was polite and courteous all the way through morning lessons, through lunch, and almost till home time. He kept a reasonable distance when looking across to steal my answers and even offered me his pencil sharpener when I snapped my point.

We only saw the *old* Adrian once the whole day. At

3:29 pm, just sixty-seconds before the end of class—so close! He whistled at Amanda and pulled one of his stupid monkey faces: pushing his ears forward with a hand on either side of his cheeks whilst making a fart sound with his mouth. She looked back at him over her shoulder and mimed the words, 'Shut up, you idiot!'

'It wasn't me, it was *him!*' The old Adrian said, pointing at me.

'God—what a hopeless dungbat that old Adrian is,' I thought, whilst packing away my pencils for another day.

But at least there's hope.

12 CYNTHIA

CYNTHIA WAS a brown lady with long plaited hair twisted into an enormous bun on top of her head. It was an architectural masterpiece. But what impressed me more was that there were no obvious signs of exterior support.

I'd seen Cynthia around the school from time to time but didn't know who she was; just some random grown-up going about their daily tasks.

Anyway, I was zipping up my pencil case and preparing for the emotional rollercoaster of morning break when she walked into the classroom and introduced herself. She told me she was from Student Services and had dropped by for a chat. This was unusual and highly suspicious. I mean—why me? And why now? Had something terrible happened to Mum? Was she here to break some bad news about Schrodinger?!

She told me to take some deep breaths because it would make me feel calm. So I did, and it worked pretty well. Although it would have been even better if she'd said exactly how many seconds I needed to breathe *in* for before breathing out again. But at least the dizziness took my mind off worrying why she'd wanted to speak to me.

Now, I don't normally like talking to people— especially if I've only just met them. But there was something I liked about Cynthia. Her sunny smile wrapped around me like a great big fluffy cloud. Somehow, I knew she was the type of person I'd be able to tell lots of private stuff to without everyone else finding out. And I'd never said that about *anyone* before, apart from Mum, Dad and Schrodinger.

After my head had stopped spinning from holding my breath for too long, she asked if I'd made any new school friends. This was especially confusing when I didn't think I had any *old* ones. But because Cynthia was so nice, I decided to have a go at answering her question.

'Well, I suppose there's Adrian Wilkes. But I wouldn't exactly use the F-R-I-E-N-D word. I certainly wouldn't want us to be like Clare Feathersdale and Amanda Goldbloom. They have sleepovers and take bites out of each other's sandwiches at lunchtime.' YUK!

'Look, I understand what you're saying, Timothy, but girls and boys have different ways of being friends with each other. You can still be friends with Adrian and not have to share sandwiches or have sleepovers. That's just how girls are. It's how they socialise. And anyway, there are different kinds of friends. Some are just the type you have in school, and others are a bit more special. The kind you invite home.'

I thought hard for a few minutes, and said: 'But how do you know which type of friend someone is?'

'Well, I suppose it depends on how you feel about that person; whether you like doing the same sort of things. You know—like hobbies.' Cynthia replied.

'GREAT! In that case, there's no way I could *ever* be friends with Adrian Wilkes because he doesn't have a clue about AstroWorld, and I have absolutely zero interest in football!'

'But you can still be friends with Adrian even though it seems you don't have much in common.'

I noticed that Cynthia's smile wasn't as big as it had been at the start of our 'chat' and that she'd folded her arms. Mum does this when she wants to change the subject. And quite honestly, I was more than happy to talk about something else. All of that stuff about having friends was beginning to get me stressed out again. So, to ease the tension, I had another look at Cynthia's twisty hairdo to see if it showed any signs of collapsing into a gigantic heap on the floor.

Incredible, I thought, it was still there—as though fixed in place with the world's strongest glue. I quickly looked away in case she caught me staring.

The next thing Cynthia asked me about was work. But I think I may have answered this in the wrong way, because I said: 'But I don't go to work, I'm still at school. Dad goes to work, and he's getting chopped.'

Cynthia's eyebrows scrunched together for a few seconds, like she wasn't sure about something, and said: 'No... sorry, I meant, how are you getting on with your schoolwork—your science lessons. I hear you're interested in astronomy?'

'Yes,' I replied, 'astronomy and physics and anything to do with Einstein. Oh... and dark matter, which I've decided to call *invisible matter* because no one can see it even though it makes up ninety per cent of the universe. I've emailed NASA and told them why *dark* should be changed to *invisible,* but they haven't got back to me about it yet. I guess they're too busy working out why the universe continues to expand faster and faster from the explosion point of the original Big Bang, when it should, in fact, be slowing down, and—'

'Okay, Timothy. TIMOTHY... okay, I get it—you can stop now, I get the picture!'

She raised the palm of her hand towards me. It reminded me of the police officer I'd seen stopping traffic on the High Street recently. They had to close the road due to an incident outside the bakery. Crusty rolls and doughnuts had been left scattered across the pavement and could not be moved until the forensics team dusted them for fingerprints. The shops were closed until the following morning. I asked Mum what had happened, but she said that some things were not for the ears of people my age. I remember wondering how old my ears would need to be before they were allowed to hear stuff that hers could?

'Anyway,' said Cynthia, 'I just wanted to let you

know that if you're feeling stressed out about anything, you can come and tell me. I'm in the Student Services office on Tuesday mornings and Friday afternoons. And don't worry, Mr Willowby knows about *EVERYTHING*.'

Now, I really wish I was one of those people who could think of good things to say *during* a conversation instead of ten hours later. But I'm not. Sometimes, the question I wished I'd asked comes along at 2 am and keeps me awake until dawn.

What exactly did Cynthia mean by, 'If I'm stressed out about anything, I should let her know?' And, 'Don't worry, Mr Willowby knows about *EVERY-THING*.' Knows about *what*, exactly?

If I was good at conversation, I would have said something like: 'Actually, Ms, there *is* something I'm worried about. I'm worried that everyone seems to know stuff that I do not. And this is *exactly* the type of thing that makes me unable to think about anything else until something even bigger comes along to stress me out!'

The bell signalling end-of-break rang, and the outside sound of noisy kids in the playground was now on the inside. The seats were filling up fast in preparation for the final lesson before lunch. It was algebra. YUK!

'What the hell happened to you? You look like you've seen a ghost!' Adrian whispered in my right ear. His hot, dungbat breath tickled the side of my face. I tried to wipe it off with my shoulder, which, as a result, also became infected by his disgusting germs.

'Don't be stupid!' I said, using my best irritated voice. 'Ghosts do not exist. It's all in the imagination. There's absolutely zero scientific evidence for the existence of paranormal activity.'

'NO, BRAINBOX! I didn't *actually* mean you've seen a ghost. It's just another way of saying you look like you're in shock. You know... like you've had some bad news or something.'

And this was when the second unusual thing happened that day. I did something I'd never done before—I actually started a conversation with someone who wasn't Mum, Dad or Schrodinger.

'Have you ever spoken to Cynthia?' I asked.

Adrian thought hard for a few seconds, like he was wondering whether it was okay to reveal an important secret.

'Yes, I have, actually. I saw her a couple of years ago when my parents got divorced and Dad went to live in Sussex with Alice. It's great there, they've got goats and chickens and a new baby who looks a bit like me—but with blond hair and blue eyes. I told you about it in the park. Remember? Cynthia said to come and see her if I wanted to talk about anything. But I said there was nothing to talk about. Anyway, why do you want to know about Cynthia?'

This was a good question. For some reason, I just couldn't remember why I'd asked him about her in the first place. And because the subject of goats seemed far more interesting I asked him about that instead.

'So... how many goats, exactly, does Alice have then? Are they kept in a barn, or are they free to roam around in the yard with the chickens? Is their milk turned into cheese, or are they mainly used to keep the grass down?'

Adrian looked confused, like he'd lost his words, or simply couldn't think of any good answers to my brilliant goat questions. I knew how he felt. I also get confused when people ask me things I don't have any expert knowledge of. My mind goes blank, and I run out of things to say.

On *small talk for beginners.com*—in the section about *how to keep a conversation going,* they advise asking follow-up questions about something the other person has just said, 'reciprocation' I think they called it. Next time I have a conversation with Adrian Wilkes, I think I'll take their advice and ask him about divorce, or Sussex, or chickens, because he obviously doesn't know much about goats.

13 BARBARA REMEMBERS

THIS WAS the day Barbara Blossom had been dreading for weeks. The day a certain brown envelope would tumble through the brass letterbox and onto the *Home Sweet Home* coconut mat by the front door.

As far as envelopes go, it was a pretty average one: oblong, with a transparent cut-out through which the names *Mr and Mrs B. Blossom* were just visible. Below, the word 'CONFIDENTIAL' was stamped diagonally in faded pillar-box red. This was indication enough that once opened, the secrets contained within might crash like a rock through the fabric of their precious domestic bliss.

Barbara stared down at the letter for a second or

two: arms folded and ashen-faced. Then returned to the kitchen hoping the letter would vanish somehow if she pretended it wasn't there. But no, there it lay unopened on the coconut mat for two hours; gathering specks of translucent dust from the shafts of sunlight streaming in through the glass-panelled door.

Barbara had let the kettle boil and cool at least five times before summoning up the courage to slice through the envelope's edge with a sharp kitchen knife. But Barbara Anne Blossom was not one to shrink from the truth—however painful it might be. She put on her reading glasses and refocused, readying herself to face the consequences of all that was printed before her.

To Barbara's surprise, the letter was disappointingly brief—to the point. As if drafted by artificial intelligence in the least possible words.

It stated:

Dear Mr and Mrs Blossom. Following Timothy's recent assessment at our clinic, we have decided on a diagnosis of ASD—Autism Spectrum Disorder. I have made

an appointment for you to visit me on June 17th at 10 am.
Please let me know if this is convenient.

Yours Sincerely

Dr Sharon Wilson

Barbara read the letter for a second time, then a third, and a fourth—just in case—then folded it back inside the envelope. She knew that life in the Blossom household would never be the same again.

The Following Week

Bert couldn't make it to the meeting to discuss Timothy's diagnosis. He was worried about the possibility of losing his job and didn't want to stir up any further trouble by taking the day off.

Barbara, pragmatic as ever—in the way mums usually are—hopped on a number 52 bus outside Greg's Groceries, and twenty-minutes later was being pointed in the direction of the child psychology department by a kindly receptionist called Mary: Patient Liaison Officer.

'Take the elevator over there to the second floor, then turn left through the double doors. You can't miss it,' she said. But Barbara shared an inconvenient trait with her son—an inability to remember directions. She'd been to the clinic before, just a few weeks earlier when Timothy had taken his tests. But still... all of those stairs and corridors; *none* of it looked even the tiniest bit familiar.

Maybe I'm a bit autistic as well? She wondered. *After all, they say these things run in families...*

Eventually, having taken an unauthorised detour through the staff canteen, she arrived at a door sign saying *Dr Sharon Wilson: PLEASE WAIT TO BE CALLED.*

'Thanks for coming in, Mrs Blossom. *Mr* Blossom couldn't make it?' She asked.

'No, sorry, Dr—trouble at work. He sends his apologies.'

'Right, well we don't have a lot of time, so we'd better make a start. As you know, we've been observing Timothy's behaviour in school for quite some time now. Cynthia from Student Services has provided some excellent feedback on how he communicates with his classmates. And his recent assessment has helped form a picture of his cognitive and emotional regulation skills. As a result, we're confident that a diagnosis of autism is appropriate.'

Barbara, who'd listened silently till now, inhaled slowly until her lungs could hold no more, then exhaled in a mighty gust to clear the tension.

'So... what exactly does all of this mean then, Dr? I mean, will he have to go to a special school or need therapy of some kind? And what *is* autism, anyway?'

'Well, basically, Mrs Blossom, autism affects a person's social and communication skills. It affects how they process information and how they relate to their surroundings. People with autism also have sensory issues. They struggle with noisy environments and bright lights and certain kinds of fabric against their skin. Some have symptoms that are much more severe than Timothy's. *They* are not able to live independent lives. But others go on to have successful careers. They even marry and have children. In my opinion, Timothy is somewhere in the middle. He has high-level skills in certain areas, but these are offset by the everyday tasks he finds more challenging. The key thing here, Mrs Blossom, is early intervention. He's only twelve, and the more help he gets to manage his social skills and emotions, the more likely it is he'll go on to live a fulfilling, independent life.'

Barbara felt the tears well up in her eyes. Big heavy tears she was determined not to release. She knew that if she lost control, for even a second, those tears would burst free into an uncontrollable flood and eat into the precious hour allocated for her appointment.

'Look, Mrs Blossom, I know you're concerned about what happens next, it's only natural, but let me reassure you, *nothing* has to change in the short term. Cynthia's built up a good relationship with Timothy. She'll keep an eye on him in school, and if we feel he's struggling, we'll think again. In the meantime, you should definitely consider discussing the diagnosis with him. After all, *he's* the one who's affected most.'

Barbara couldn't remember leaving Dr Wilson's office *or* descending to the ground floor in a silver elevator that smelled of disinfectant. She climbed aboard the 52 bus to East Winslow High Street without even checking the number. But she may just as easily have stepped onto a 72 by mistake and ended up in Drayton, six miles in the opposite direction. Or been found wandering the AstroWorld car park, dazed and confused, having unwittingly ridden a number 103 to West Cranford. Barbara Blossom was aware of nothing. Only the words of Dr Sharon Wilson, the woman who'd made everything so painfully, so devastatingly, so finally, official.

14 THE DAY I FOUND OUT

Sunday

MUM AND DAD had just done the annual mega-tidy-up, and the house smelled fresher than a forest in spring. But as I lay on my bed with the scent of pine and honeysuckle drifting under my door, I could not have known that soon I would be a *new* Timothy: changed yet unchanged. A version of me that was entirely different, yet virtually indistinguishable from the one I'd known for twelve years, six months, and thirty-two days.

～

I'd spent the morning relaxing in my room with the sound of waves rising and falling through my new noise-cancelling headphones. Meanwhile, Schrodinger was busy splashing around in his tank, practising his impressive backstroke.

The surf-topped saltwater spray in my ears was so loud I didn't hear Mum come in. She tapped me on the shoulder and gestured that I should come downstairs. So I turned off the ocean and gave Schrodinger a double thumbs-up for the excellent demonstration of goldfish backstroke. He floated sideways for a second or two without gulping—code for, 'Well if you think *that* was good, you'll be amazed when I show you my dolphin impression!' I could have sworn I saw his tiny teeth glisten when his mouth widened into an orange U-shape.

I followed Mum downstairs and made a mental note that later I would do some research into whether goldfish smile. But I wouldn't let Schrodinger know what I was doing. He worries when I get obsessed by stuff that most people would neither think of nor care about.

Dad was already sitting in his armchair by the window when I sunk down onto the old green couch that Mum had been trying to get rid of for years.

'That thing's like a McDonald's for moths!' She'd say—hoping Dad would take the hint and have it hauled away in a garbage truck.

'Alright, Love, I'll sort it out on the weekend,' he'd say from behind the *Gazette's* oversized pages. But I don't think he ever will.

In fact, now I think about it, it wasn't unreasonable to think that Dad didn't actually exist above the waist. Most of the time, all anyone could see below that newspaper was a pair of legs protruding downwards into a pair of comfy slippers.

But today was different. There he was, in full view; his *Gazette* folded neatly on the side, waiting for Mum to begin the conversation.

'Now, Timothy, there's something very important Dad and I need to tell you. So I want you to concentrate *really* hard and not drift off. You may not understand everything we're going to say, but I just want to let you know that Dad and I are here to help, and if you ever want to talk about the thing I'm going to tell you, then—'

'FOR GOD'S SAKE BARBARA... CAN'T YOU

JUST GET ON WITH IT?! THE BOY'S AUTISTIC HE'S NOT STUPID... OOPS—!'

Mum looked at Dad in a really bad way. Like she was so angry she was going to cry, or maybe even ask for a divorce.

'You've really spoilt things, Bert. I've been planning my little speech for days, and now you, you and that great big mouth of yours have messed the whole thing up. WELL THANK YOU *VERY* MUCH INDEED!'

'Sorry, Love,' Dad said, hoping that Mum would like him again as soon as possible. 'It's just that... well, sometimes—if you don't mind me saying—you have a habit of turning the tiniest of molehills into the mightiest of mountains. He's autistic that's all. Lots of kids are autistic. He'll grow out of it.'

'YOU'VE DONE IT *AGAIN,* BERT! You've said *that* word, the 'A-word.' The word we weren't going to mention just yet!'

'But if we don't mention *that* word, how will he ever know what we're talking about?' Dad fired back, hoping not to make Mum angry again.

I was very, *very* confused by this point. For starters, why was Dad talking about molehills and mountains? The only thing around here that may have looked like a mountain to a mole was the grassy slope in the park that kids slid down when it snowed, but to a human, *that* barely even qualified as a hill!

Mum looked at me and took the deepest breath I'd ever seen a person take, and said: 'Do you remember those tests you had a couple of months ago? The ones I said were to find out how brainy you are? Well... they sort of were—to see how brainy you are. And we found out that you are, indeed, extremely brainy, but in a very special way. It turns out that you have something called—'

Mum stopped talking and cleared her throat.

'What your mum is trying to say, Timothy, is that you have something called ASD—autism spectrum disorder. That letter, the one you were trying to get a peek at a few weeks ago, was from the psychologist who did the tests. She said that some of your results were way above average for your age. "Astonishing" was the *actual* word she used. But in some of the other tests... well, let's just say you didn't do quite so well.'

Now I was more confused than ever.

Was I brainy or not? Am I ill? And if I am, is it catching? Will it mean surgery? Will I have to spend weeks recovering in hospital with wires sticking out from everywhere? The questions were exploding in my head like fireworks on November 5th, and I couldn't make them stop.

Mum must have also heard the fireworks because she said: 'No, Timothy, you're not ill, you just see things differently to other people. The *thing* you have explains why you're so incredibly brilliant at astronomy and physics, but also why you misunderstand simple instructions sometimes. It's why you like to wear your socks inside out, and why you prefer your own company. It explains why you don't like loud noises, and why you hate in-between days that are neither hot nor cold, winter or summer—'

Then Mum stopped talking again and poured another cup of tea. She looked at Dad to see if he had anything vaguely useful to add, and then at me in case I had any follow-up questions. There were at least a million things I wanted to ask, but for some reason, I could not turn a single thought into words. So, instead, I sat silently on the old green couch counting the moth holes, wondering if Dad ever would find the time to drag it off to the recycling centre.

～

I wasn't sure how I felt about what Mum and Dad had told me. Mainly because I didn't understand most of it. Something about 'thinking differently to other people' and 'having a condition but not being ill.' And because of it, I'm extremely clever and not at all clever at the same time. And that it's a disorder which also has its good points and sort of rhymes with ballistic *(the motion of objects influenced by the force of gravity)*. But it also has another name that almost rhymes with prism *(a polyhedron with two parallel surfaces whose lateral faces are parallelograms)*.

I suppose I was quite glad in a way that being my type of different had an official name. And that my 'unique wiring' made me so incredibly special—even if it *did* make me sound like a cyborg in a Hollywood blockbuster.

But *special* can also mean *weird*. And when you're twelve, being weird is the last thing anyone wants to be. Especially in school when everyone's trying so hard to fit in.

I decided that, for now, the 'A-word' would remain a well-kept secret. Locked firmly inside the Blossom family circle of trust, to be spoken of only by Mum, Dad, Schrodinger and me.

15 THE 'A-WORD'

I CAME down to breakfast on my first 'A-word' morning expecting the world would be changed beyond all recognition. But no, the table was strewn with the usual breakfast-time clutter of jam and marmalade jars, teapots, crumb-filled plates and butter knives. A familiar plume of hot-milk steam rose from my AstroWorld space mug and headed skywards as it always does towards the white-washed ceiling. There was not a single shred of evidence to suggest that the world had become even the tiniest bit different to the one I'd been used to before I found out I had the 'A-word.'

In fact, I was beginning to wonder if that 'A-word'

conversation had really happened. Perhaps I'd dreamt the whole thing.

But one thing *was* different: Mum was a lot quieter than usual. She rinsed the dishes and stacked them into a neat pile on the side, drying her hands on the *I Heart USA* towel Frank and Leslie brought back from Miami. She came over and sat down just a bit too close for my liking, so I squeaked my chair sideways a few inches against the ceramic floor tiles to get some breathing space.

'So, Timothy, how do you feel about what Dad and I told you yesterday?'

If I could've worked out how to reply, my answers would have included the words *embarrassed* and *scared*. *Embarrassed*, because I was now officially the most different kid in my class. And *scared* because I didn't know what having the 'A-word' actually meant.

Autism, or the 'A-word' as I prefer to call it, used to be one of those words that pass in through one ear and straight out through the other. It gets talked about at school sometimes, usually when Highcrest have one of their incredibly boring *diversity-awareness-days*.

Experts come in to speak about disability, and racism, and other dull but important stuff. We write poems about how everyone has a special gift, and how we are all equal but different—the same, yet totally unique. Wow, talk about confusing!

But the worst part is when you have to stand up and read your poem out loud. And when you're finished, the whole class applauds like you're a rock star or something.

Maybe it's just me, but it all seems kind of fake. As though a bunch of well-meaning adults got together in the staff room and decided how kids should think about everything. I agree that being nice to each other is a good thing, but it can't possibly be true that *everyone* has a special gift to share with the world. I sit next to Adrian Wilkes—remember? And he doesn't appear to have a talent for *anything*. Not unless being the most annoying excuse for a human on the entire planet makes him unique and special. Although, now I think about it, I suppose it does, in a funny kind of not very good way.

But anyway, this was a day for thinking exclusively about the 'A-word'—not that skunk-breath-lizard-wart Wilkes. So, I brought my thoughts back to what Mum and Dad had told me about my 'special wiring' and thought about nothing else until bedtime, other than a few related topics, such as hating Sunday evenings, litterbugs and escalators.

My very first 'A-word' journey to school was surprisingly uneventful. I tiptoed past Trevor, who was, as usual, snoozing just inside the neighbour's garden gate. He opened half a sleepy eye. 'GRRR' he growled, without moving a single hairy muscle, then fell silent again like a fat, furry rug.

As I made my way along Eaton Drive, I noticed how strangely familiar everything seemed: the houses, the trees, the red postbox on the corner, even that rusty old lamp post with a weather-beaten picture of a missing cat called *Misty* stuck on the side.

Somehow, I thought my earth-shattering 'A-word' news would have transformed the entire area into a post-apocalyptic vision of 'A-word' hell. The streets would be lined with flesh-eating zombies. They'd point and mock with fingers twisted by gangrenous sludge. Drool, brown and acidic, would drip from their maggot-eaten mouths:

'A-WORD KID... A-WORD KID... WE'RE

COMING TO GET YOU. A-WORD KID!' They'd sneer and snarl.

Well, okay, so I may be exaggerating a bit. I didn't really think flesh-eating zombies would follow me to school. But I did think that some of the neighbours would say, 'Look, there's that officially different kid from 47 Eaton Drive.' And I did think that Adrian Wilkes would refuse to sit next to me in class, and that no one would volunteer to take his place. But no, just the usual, 'OY, BRAINBOX, WANNA SEE MY BRUISE?!'

And you know what? For once, just once, I was actually quite pleased to hear Adrian make one of his stupid comments. It was like old times—before I discovered I was one of those kids they talk about on diversity days. One of those 'uniquely gifted' kids who are 'equal, yet different.' The type everyone makes allowances for. The type who gets a medal and a round of applause for coming last in the sports day egg and spoon race.

How fake and embarrassing is *that?!*

16 BERT BLOSSOM

Bert

ALL YOU HEAR about these days is disability this and disability that. Everyone seems to have an 'ism' of some description. But where's it all come from? We never had autism or dyslexia or ADHD or anything like that when I was growing up. When I was a lad, in school, there were the 'good kids' who always did well in their exams, and the 'naughty kids' who the teacher said would probably end up in prison. Then there were the barely average kids, like me, whose prospects were somewhere in the middle.

I was more of a practical, hands-on type and grew up thinking books were for the clever kids with posh parents. Kids like me and Alf—well, we spent more time kicking footballs around in the street than we ever did studying. But secretly, I wanted to be more like the clever kids. The type destined for university and a well-paid job in the city. The problem was, I could read a sentence five-times over, then five-times over again, and still be none the wiser. Either the words wouldn't go 'in' in the first place, or I'd forget each one in a heartbeat.

The teachers called me lazy, stupid, and slow because I couldn't read as quickly as some of the others. But, you know what? Show me a broken motorbike engine when I was sixteen and I'd have it fixed within the hour. And that's how I got into engineering. I left school without a single qualification to my name and went straight into an apprenticeship with *KPW Automation.* And I haven't looked back since. I suppose you could say I've developed my own way of doing things—of getting by. Although, I must admit, all of this new computer technology has left me feeling a bit prehistoric. Back in the good old days, it took four of us to push a row of buttons and crank some hefty handles. But now, a single, fresh-out-of-uni-kid with a degree in performing arts can operate a factory full of machines with the click of a plastic mouse. Where's the skill in that, I ask? It's little wonder KPW are talking about cutting staff and replacing them with minimum-wage button-pushers.

Don't get me wrong; I don't want to give the impression that I'm stuck in my ways, and I'm certainly not illiterate. I can read a newspaper well enough and I've always been a whizz with numbers. It's just that I'm always reading things wrong; thinking a headline in the Gazette means one thing when it really means something else. Barbara's always saying, 'Oh, for God's sake, Bert, you're just like Timothy—the way you see things.' And I suppose she's right. I do see things a bit off-centre, off-key, wide of the mark. It's just the way my brain works —or *DOESN'T!* As she keeps reminding me.

Still, I've done alright, I suppose. I've always worked hard. You know—tried to do my best.

I must admit, though, it's not easy bringing up a boy like Timothy. To say he's got his challenges would be the understatement of the century. He's calm one minute and screaming at the top of his voice the next; throwing anything he can get his hands on across the room when his emotions get the better of him. It wasn't so bad when he was younger, and we had a bit more control. But he's almost as tall as Barbara now.

God knows how we'll handle him when he's a strapping seventeen-year-old.

I haven't said this to Barbara, but sometimes I think we should consider getting him into one of those supported-living places. After all, we're not getting any younger. We need to start planning for the future. I mean, what will happen when he leaves school? How can he ever hope to hold down a steady job? Everything has to be so perfect around him: the spaces between the pencils on his homework desk, the lighting, the sounds, the smells, the people, the temperature, the texture of his clothes. No one would employ such a fussy person—not in a million years.

But the one thing I just can't seem to get my head around is how he can be so incredibly smart one moment, and so utterly incapable of doing the most basic of things the next. I mean, most of the time I haven't got a clue what he's talking about when he's going on about all of that science stuff, yet the boy can't even dress himself or run a bath. What will happen when he meets a girl and gets married? Who will knot his tie and button his shirt each morning? Who will cut the edges off his bread and take the hard bits out of his orange juice? Who'd want a husband that throws a hissy fit because his cabbage touched a roast potato?

Quite frankly, what with all the trouble at work and worrying about Timothy's future—I feel like locking myself in the garden shed and never coming out!

I'd never say this to Barbara, but sometimes I wish I could be a teenager again. Those were the days. Young, free and single, without a care in the world.

Life was so simple back then....

17   THE PRICE OF CHANGE

'HOW MUCH DID this lot cost then?' The palm of Bert's hand was pushed flat and hard against his worried brow. He'd returned home from work to find the coffee table stacked higher than Waterstones with books on how to parent a child with autism.

'WHAT THE—!'

A quick scan around the kitchen revealed multi-coloured post-it notes with instructions stuck to every door, window frame, work surface and appliance. There wasn't a single switch without information on how to click on and how to click off. There wasn't a tap without a diagram indicating which way to turn for hot, cold, faster and slower.

'What the hell is going on, Barbara? You've practically redecorated the place!'

'Oh, *do* calm down, Bert, you'll have a heart attack if you carry on like this!' She folded her arms and prepared to defend her position: 'If you'd bothered to read the information leaflets I brought home from Dr Wilson's office the other day, you'd know that children with autism need prompting. She recommends we use visual aids like pictures with clear instructions. It helps them process information and remember things. I want to make things as easy for Timothy as possible.'

Barbara's reasoning calmed Bert for a few seconds until he noticed, in the corner of the living room by the cheese plant, a large unopened box with the words, *Evans Electricals,* stamped on the side in a thick black font. Again, Bert's forehead erupted into long fleshy furrows at the thought of yet more unexpected expense.

'Don't panic, Bert, they're only light bulbs, low-powered ones. They were delivered today whilst you were at work. I read that autistic children hate bright lights and loud noise. So, from now on, this house will be an oasis of serenity. An environmentally friendly, low-arousal space where Timothy—AND

YOU, by the looks of things—can retreat from the stress and strain of daily life.'

Bert shook his head slowly in disbelief, clutching at his wallet through the fabric of his jacket.

'Crikey, Barbara, you sound like you've swallowed a medical dictionary. All you talk about these days is autism this, and autism that. You're making the boy think there's something wrong with him. He's just a bit different—a bit quirky, that's all. He hasn't got a disease or grown another leg. He's just *Timothy*. The same Timothy he's always been. You can't keep him wrapped up in cotton wool for the rest of his life. It's a dog-eat-dog world out there. How's he ever going to learn to look after himself with you mollycoddling him the whole time?'

MOLLYCODDLING?! I wondered from my vantage point on the hall staircase. Is that even a real word?

I'd been sitting there the whole time, hoping I wouldn't get caught eavesdropping again by Dad. He said that spying on other people's conversations is an unhealthy pastime. And for the record, I agree, but how else am I supposed to find stuff out around here? No one tells me *ANYTHING!*

He was right about one thing though, there were

stickers and laminated pictures with instructions all over the house. On the wall behind the toaster, a photo showed a slice of burnt bread leaping into the air. Another, on the wall tiles behind the sink, was of water pouring from a tap; cartoon hands grasped at a slippery bar of soap. Even the toilet bowl had a water-proof target stuck to the bottom. The words 'PEE HERE' were written on it. In my opinion, the toilet one was secretly meant for Dad. *My* aim is truer than a laser-guided missile!

Mum even bought a brand new state-of-the-art doorbell: *The Easy Ring 5000*. It was the only one of its type in East Winslow. I know this because I took a picture of every single doorbell on the way home from school. That evening I analysed the images in my computer, and not one came close to matching ours in design, ergonomics, and technology. Mum had definitely done her homework and picked a winner. To be honest, I was more than happy to see the back of that old Big Ben of a doorbell. The new one chimes softer than a bell tree in heaven. For this, I am truly grateful.

But as for all the other changes? Like the new light bulbs that keep the house in a state of constant gloom? I kept thinking *WOW! Mum is totally obsessed with all of this 'A-word' stuff.* But then I felt guilty and upset because she'd worked so hard to make my life as stress-free as possible. I almost cried when Dad made fun of her because she'd bothered learning all of those complicated '*A-word*' words like neurotypical, theory of mind, executive functioning, developmental delay and emotional regulation.

'What are you—a psychologist?!' I heard Dad say to her the other day.

'NO!' She replied. 'BUT AT LEAST I'M NOT A USELESS, GOOD-FOR-NOTHING, DISINTER-ESTED LUMP OF GRUMPY OLD LARD LIKE YOU!'

She slammed the kitchen door behind her with such force the antique picture of a Farmhouse in Devon fell from the wall and smashed into a thousand tiny pieces. I was convinced that Mum and Dad would never speak to each other again. I ran up to my room and let the tears out for eleven minutes and fourteen seconds. I spent a further eighteen minutes counting the planets on my AstroWorld wallpaper. This calmed me down for a while, but it couldn't take away the sadness.

'What are we going to do *now*, Schrodinger? Everything's changing so fast. I don't know who I am anymore. Mum and Dad's marriage is over, and I'll probably end up in a hostel for homeless kids that doesn't allow pets. I may never see you again! Will life *ever* get back to normal?'

Schrodinger blew four larger than average bubbles—code for, 'WOW! THIS IS A REALLY BAD SITUATION, but don't worry, things always turn out for the best in the end.' He stared knowingly, calmly at me through the glass. Somehow, I knew he understood. But then... he always does; my best friend, Schrody.

18 MY FIRST 'A-WORD' BIRTHDAY

'HAPPY SPECIAL THIRTEENTH BIRTHDAY!'

My bedroom door practically flew off its hinges and in barged Mum with my birthday breakfast. She was right, this was a special day. 'One of a kind,' I think she called it. But I wasn't exactly sure if it was one of a *good* kind, or one of a kind filled with tons of terrible stuff that would make me want to be twelve again.

It was my first ever 'A-word' birthday, and I was now officially a teenager; even though Mum had been saying I was practically one for weeks—months, in fact. But then she'll go on about how I should never wish my life away by wanting Monday mornings to be Friday afternoons. I mean, how hypocritical is *that*?

The implications of passing the childhood halfway mark was not something I'd given much thought to before. For the first time in my life, I could really understand why old people shake their heads and say, 'Where on God's green earth did the years go?' Although, why old people describe the world like this is a mystery. There's nothing 'green' about most of it. From space, it looks mainly blueish and fluffy white. Anyhow, today was the day I realised that, for the next seven years, my age would have *T-E-E-N* on the end—something I'd not considered yesterday when I was twelve and still had my whole life ahead of me.

According to Mum, this was also supposed to be a happy day. A day of celebration, of receiving presents and eating too much chocolate. The day by which my old babyish toys should have been given to the charity shop in the High Street to make way for a bunch of new stuff that matched my age. Schrodinger had gulped nervously when he heard Mum say all of my old things should be dispensed with.

'Don't worry, Schrody,' I said, after she'd left the room, 'I don't think she was talking about you.'

He flipped over onto his back and drifted casually for a while—relieved.

This year, my birthday fell on a Saturday. I was more than happy about this even though it meant breaking the rule that states we should only visit AstroWorld on Sundays when it's not so busy.

Last year, when my birthday fell on a school day, Mum got me into class extra early and left an enormous chocolate cake on Mr Willowby's desk. It had my name and age stamped on the top in blue icing. Twelve rocket-shaped candles pointed skywards. At break time, everyone gathered around Mr Willowby's desk to sing happy birthday and receive a fat crumbly slice in a tissue. How embarrassing! And then, to make matters worse, Adrian thought it would be fun to blow out *my* candles with *his* hot slimy breath before I had a chance to. There was no way I was going to eat any birthday cake after that. YUK! No surprise then, when half the class went down with an unusually potent strain of stomach bug. Coincidence or *what*?

Anyway, according to my calculations, I wouldn't need to endure another school-day-birthday-celebration for at least another three years. Not if I take holidays, weekends, and the sick days I'm planning to take off, into account. By then I'll be practically an adult and more able to cope with things.

This year, Mum pinned a colour-coded list of birthday activities to the corkboard organiser by the cooker. It was smeared with dried grease where she'd tried to clean it. Apparently, Dad's sausages had exploded in the pan at breakfast. Dribbles of cold fat still clung to its laminated surface.

I could just make out the following:

- 10 am—receive presents
- 11 am—one hour's quality time with Schrodinger
- Noon—birthday lunch
- 1:47 pm—catch the train from East Winslow
- 2:29 pm—arrive at West Cranford
- 3:04 pm—enter AstroWorld

This was as far as Mum had got with the list. She said it was always good to leave a space for the unexpected. Because, 'One never knows what brilliant, life-changing surprises might happen.'

But I thought she knew I hated 'brilliant, life-changing surprises,' and that I certainly didn't want any happening on my birthday. Not unless they were totally planned, brilliant, life-changing surprises approved by me at least three days in advance.

Mum eventually gave in and added a few extra things to the itinerary:

- 5:30 pm—return home
- 6:30 pm—special birthday dinner
- 9:30 pm—bed

Okay, so I don't think she gave as much thought to the evening's birthday activities as she might have done, but at least I had something to work with.

The first thing Dad said to me today was the same thing he's said every single birthday since I learnt to speak. It's become like this weird comedy sketch that always makes me cringe. He'll start with: 'So—how does it feel to be a year older then?'

Then I'll say: 'I feel the same as I did yesterday.'

Then he'll say: '*Son*—you're as old as you feel. And when you get to our age, you won't feel a blimmin thing. Isn't that right, Barbara?'

Then Mum will say: 'Speak for yourself, you silly old fool!' She'll roll her eyes and giggle just enough to humour him.

This year, after Dad had completed his annual comedy routine and disappeared back behind the enormous pages of *The East Winslow Gazette,* Mum swapped her *pretending-to-be-amused* face for one that was no longer squeezing out a smile.

'So, seriously, Timmy, how *do* you feel about being thirteen? Now that you've reached such an important milestone in your life?'

I thought about milestones for a few seconds and said, 'I don't know, Mum. You know I can't answer questions like that.'

The image of a concrete post by the side of a road inscribed with the words *Timothy Blossom—age thir-*

teen, flashed through my mind. Carved arrows pointed in different directions: to my past, my present, and my future. I wanted to follow the arrow that said 'my past' because it was the direction that looked safest. After all, no one can possibly know the future because it hasn't happened yet, and the present doesn't exist either, because the moment it happens it's already behind you. So, when you think about it, the past is all we have....

I must have fallen into one of my deep moments when I forget that someone's waiting for an answer. I snapped back into the moment that had already become the past and saw that Mum's face was shaped in a way that meant she had lots of jumbled up thoughts bouncing around all over the place. And that's exactly how I felt about being thirteen—all jumbled up.

My first 'A-word' birthday had been comfortingly uneventful. As though whoever was in charge of birthdays had, as a special treat, granted me an anniversary of my birth that was almost entirely predictable. A day of stress-free perfection, clouded only by the late arrival of the 13:47 following a signal failure at Heatherbridge. This meant that by the time our train arrived to take us to West Cranford—the closest stop to AstroWorld—there were twice as many commuters waiting on the platform as there should have been. And as far as I'm concerned, twice as many commuters means twice the amount of things to worry about:

What will happen if everyone pushes past me to get on the train? What will happen if we don't get a seat? What will happen if I have to sit next to someone I don't like the look of? What will I do if someone starts having a loud conversation on their phone?

Dad made sure I got a window seat and sat next to me in case a stranger tried to sit there; then he handed me my noise-cancelling headphones. The sound of waves crashing on a faraway shore began to fill my ears and comfort my thoughts. I turned the volume up as loud as it would go and closed my eyes until I was no longer on a train. Instead, I was relaxing on a beach, massaged by a warm Cornish breeze.

Ahh... Seagulls hanging high in the salt sea air. Fish, chips and mushy peas on a cod-shaped plate in the café by the harbour. That sunny afternoon we explored rock pools for shells to put in Schrodinger's tank. Last year's holiday with Mum and Dad in St Ives. The week I'd wished would never end and prayed would come again soon—

I felt a hand on my shoulder, it was Dad. 'Wake up, sleepyhead! We're almost at West Cranford.'

For some reason, I wasn't in an AstroWorld mood that day. After a quick browse around the space-helmet department, Dad and I had a cup of hot chocolate in the Stargazer Café and left without buying anything. I guess the stress of being thirteen was beginning to catch up with me. That's what happens when you get older. You hit 'milestones' as Mum puts it and suddenly there's all of this extra stuff to worry about. Like growing out of your favourite clothes and finding new ones that don't itch.

Yesterday, when I was only twelve, the future was but a distant horizon. Today, I have the horrible feeling that thirteen will become seventeen, then twenty-one, then thirty-three. By then, Mum and Dad will be old and frail. Who will look after me and Schrodinger? Who will scrape the algae from his tank and cut the crusts from my bread?

Today, the future is laughing at me from a scary white clown face with big red lips, and I can't laugh back.

I'm scared, Mum, that's how I honestly feel about being thirteen—I'm really, *really* scared.

19 A VERY BIG DAY

7:01 am

I WOKE up wishing the world beyond my bedroom had ceased to exist. Gone like some horrible dream in the night. From below the covers I heard the door creak open—three soft footsteps were followed by a pause.

'I want to apologise for losing my temper last night. I promise it won't happen again.' Mum's warm tone floated towards my ears and offered the tiniest sign of hope that the Blossoms may yet survive. And that Dad wouldn't go off and meet someone like Adrian's stepmother, Alice, who breeds goats in Sussex.

Mum may have cheered me up a bit, but there

were still a few important things I needed to know. 'Where will me and Schrodinger live when you and Dad get divorced?' I asked.

'WHAT—DIVORCED?! What in the world makes you think your father and I are getting divorced?'

'Well, it's obvious, isn't it? You slammed the door so hard last night, the whole house shook.'

'Don't be silly, your father and I are not getting divorced. We just had a disagreement, that's all. *His* problem is that he doesn't like to be proved wrong. It will all blow over in a couple of days when he realises that I was right all along. Now, hurry up and get ready for school. It's a big day today; we don't want to be late, do we now?'

By the way, I really don't know why Mum always says, 'We' and 'Our' when she wants me to do something I don't particularly want to do. She'll say, 'Let's finish *our* homework, shall *we?*' Then she'll disappear into the kitchen to read a magazine on gardening, or call Leslie for a chat. Or she'll say, 'Let's tidy *our* room, shall *we?*' Then she'll sneak out and leave me and Schrodinger to do all the work.

But Mum was right about one thing. Today was, without a shadow of a doubt, going to be a big day. An enormous day, in fact. Technically, of course, it's not possible to measure the size of a day, so I'll rephrase this to, today is going to be a horrendously stressed out, belly-aching, headache-inducing kind of day. Furthermore, it should be totally against my human rights to suffer a twenty-four-hour stretch of such disgustingly terrible time.

And speaking of time: if I could travel back to last Saturday, I'd hide Mum's keys so she couldn't leave the house to go shopping. Unfortunately, she'd bumped into Sue Wilkes (Adrian's mother) in that new superstore a couple of miles away. Mum had been browsing there for gluten-free food because she'd read somewhere that some 'A-word' kids have a thing called *gluten intolerance*. Mum and Mrs Wilkes ended up having this great big conversation about diet, and how food can affect how we feel, and how, apparently, 'we are what we eat.' This is a pretty weird concept because we always have sausages and beans for supper on Fridays. So just *what*, exactly, does that make me?

Anyway, during the conversation, Sue Wilkes suggested that I go over to her place with Adrian after school one day for tea. And for some reason, Mum stupidly agreed without asking me first. And now, here I am, on the morning of the dreaded 'Adrian day' wishing I'd never been born.

Adrian was late for school that morning, and I know it sounds bad, but I was hoping that he'd stayed home because he had a really bad cold, or maybe chicken-pox. Or that he'd been abducted by aliens from one of those pathetic UFO conspiracy videos he watches on the internet. *That* would be even more brilliant! Mr Willowby would probably pull me aside at lunchtime to break the news of Adrian's abduction to a faraway galaxy. I'd pretend to be sad, but inside I'd be happy because I'd get to spend a normal evening at home with Mum, Dad, and Schrodinger.

But just as I was beginning to think this may not be such a bad day after all, the classroom door crashed open and in fell Adrian-dungbat-worsel-toad-Wilkes; the contents of his backpack scattered as he landed spread-eagled on the floor.

'Ouch, that *really* hurt!' He groaned to muted giggles from around the room.

'YOU'RE LATE, WILKES!' Mr Willowby bellowed.

'Yes, I know, sorry, Sir, it won't happen again.'

Adrian climbed slowly to his feet. 'I er—I got lost on the way, and my bus was late, and I forgot my travel pass, and my lunch, and my homework, and I stepped in dog mess so I had to stop and scrape it off, and I thought it was Sunday so I didn't get up on time, and...'

On and on he went like an avalanche of pathetic drivel. I'd never heard such a terrible collection of excuses for being late. Even by HIS incredibly low standards they were rubbish.

Mr Willowby shook his head in disgust and returned to the pile of unmarked homework on his desk.

'You still coming over to my place tonight?' Adrian asked, dumping his backpack clumsily onto the table. This forced my carefully arranged colouring pencils to pile up on top of each other until there was no longer a one-centimetre gap between each one.

'NO!' I screamed, trying to reposition my pencils into non-touching lines. I began rocking backwards and forwards, and crying, and banging my fist on the table. Clare and Amanda, and all the other kids whose names I'd never bothered learning, turned to witness my embarrassing meltdown. But in that moment I was too far gone to care. The next thing I knew, Cynthia was standing over me with a glass of water, asking if I needed some quiet time.

She led me to a room at the far end of the main corridor next to headteacher Ellen Ford's office. On the door, a sign said: 'STUDENT SERVICES— PLEASE KNOCK BEFORE ENTERING,' but we ignored it and went straight in.

Cynthia's office had a view of the playground I'd not seen before. Below was a flat roof where at least a dozen footballs had become lodged and unreachable, deflated and discoloured; their owners probably long-gone from Highcrest Manor.

Inside, a poster on the wall featured a young boy who looked sad. He was alone, watching the rain through a misty window. Below, helpline numbers offered confidential advice and support. Another poster was about bullying. A teenager was cowering; circled by an angry pack of wolves. The headline read, 'IT'S TIME TO BITE BACK!' It reminded me of a nightmare I once had, so I couldn't look at it for long.

Further along the wall, holiday snaps were stuck

to a shiny whiteboard. In one of them, Cynthia was sipping a blue drink through a stripy straw that matched her fingernails. She wore sunglasses and a flowery sombrero. The buildings in the background looked white-hot like the ones I'd seen in Spain. Mum and Dad took me there once when I was five. We spent a week on the Costa del Sol. I made sand-castles on the beach and got sunburnt. That's all I have to say about Spain. Personally, I prefer Cornwall. In summer there's just the right amount of heat, and in winter you can walk for miles along a sandy beach without seeing anyone.

'So, would you like to talk about what just happened in class, Timothy?'

Cynthia's voice suddenly appeared in my ears, reminding me that I was in her office. And because she seemed so nice and friendly, I told her every single tiny detail. I told her about all the 'A-word' stuff that was going on at home, and how the *Farmhouse in Devon* picture had smashed on the floor after Mum got angry and slammed the door. Then I told her about Schrodinger and how I hate being called *Timmy*. Then I talked about how extra-stressed-out I felt because I was supposed to be going home with Adrian Wilkes after school that day. I must have rambled on for ages; I'd completely forgotten that Cynthia was even in the room!

She cleared her throat—the way people often do when they want me to stop talking—and said, 'You should definitely go to Adrian's house, just for an hour or two. And if you don't like it there, you can always call Mum to pick you up early. After all, Eaton Drive is only a few streets away. It'll be fun.'

I remember thinking that if 'fun' was a place, it would be at least ten trillion light-years away from Adrian's house. But, because Cynthia had such a friendly smile, and such perfectly painted star signs embossed in silver on her sky-tinted fingernails, I agreed to go. But only if Mum remained on standby with her phone fully charged.

'It's a deal!' Cynthia said, giving me a high-five and promising to call Mum with instructions to prepare for an emergency evacuation from Adrian's if the need should arise. It was then I decided to add Cynthia to my *most trusted* list when I got home. It's taped to the back of my bedroom door next to all the other lists. There aren't many people on my *most trusted* list—just three, actually, and they're all Blossoms. Mum and Schrodinger are currently in joint first place, and then comes Dad. *His* name is always written in pencil because sometimes I have to demote him even further down than being last. And now there's 'Cynthia' scrawled in shades of blue crayon to match her fingernails. *Erasable* blue crayon—just in case.

20 ADRIAN'S HOUSE

I USUALLY TURN *RIGHT* through the playground gate when I leave school at 3:30 pm each day. My journey takes me past the entrance to Sparrow Hill Park where the 'normal' boys—as Dad puts it—play football on Sunday mornings. Next to it is an old church with stained-glass windows and a bell that hasn't chimed since 1978. Everyone says the place is haunted, but in my opinion, the supernatural is for bored people with nothing better to think about. Although I must admit, I normally cross over to the other side of the street when it's Halloween—just in case.

I haven't calculated exactly how many times I've

been that way before, but it's a route I know so well, that once I even attempted to walk home with my eyes closed. It was going well until Mum decided to let go of my hand to answer her phone!

But anyway, today was different, I was doing the *unbelievable*; I was going to Adrian's place. I followed him out of the school gate and turned *left* along the pavement instead. This was a journey into uncharted territory, a route I had not travelled, and each step was leading me deeper into the unknown.

I could almost hear my heart pound above the traffic as we turned the corner into the 'bad' end of the High Street. It was the part Dad says was once like a picturesque village, but now he avoids it like the plague. Well, there may not have been diseased bodies lying by the side of the road crawling with maggots and flies, but it was certainly a good deal scruffier than I could have imagined.

On the other side of the street, next to the charity shop, kids in burgundy jackets and grey trousers were eating from boxes outside the Dixie Chicken take-away. One of them dropped a cola-can and crushed it underfoot. Another threw his leftovers over his shoulder; it landed on the pavement and was quickly swept away on a gust of dirty air.

'Stop staring at them!' Adrian said, elbowing me in the side. 'They're from Haversdale Academy. You don't want to mess with that lot. Just keep walking.'

I remained silent and continued along the High Street, fixing my gaze instead on the *Megasave* where Mum used to buy milk and bread; before, according to Dad, the area became a hub for undesirables who hang around outside betting shops all day, whistling at girls and asking passers-by for money.

Mum, who prefers to see the best in people, thought Dad was being mean and said:

'Let he who is without sin cast the first stone.'

Personally, I think Mum should speak in a way we can *all* understand—otherwise, what's the point?

Dad was right about the filthy bus shelter, though. It was covered in the same swirly shapes that had been popping up all over the neighbourhood recently. It's like a bunch of invisible teenage hooligans stalk the streets at night, spraying dustbins, and shop windows, and trees, and trains.

Some of their 'artwork' is even on the sides of buildings where it's impossible to reach unless you're dangling from a helicopter by a rope. I didn't actually see any, but I bet there were even a few graffiti-covered cats and dogs roaming the mean streets of East Winslow Town Centre.

Anyway, as Adrian and I passed the bus shelter, I noticed the side-panel was missing. Its shattered glass had been swept into the gutter. I felt sorry for the old lady waiting for the number 27 to Hollywell Lane. I bet *she* remembers the good old days. We both jumped when a motorbike roared past like an angry, black metal lion. Surely there must be a law against such violently intrusive noise levels on the public highway? But it didn't seem to bother Adrian. I guess his ears are not as sensitive as mine.

Now, I don't know if the pavements in East Winslow are wonky in my favour, but Adrian appeared to be at least an inch shorter than I'd imagined. Strange, considering his birthday was before mine, thus making him slightly older. I also noticed a small, jagged scar above his left eyebrow, and that his nose was splattered with pale freckles. It's funny how you can sit next to someone for two years without really looking at them.

'So, what's your favourite football team, then?' He asked for no apparent reason.

'I don't like football,' I replied.

'Okay then,' he said, 'do you have a favourite food?'

I thought this was getting just a little too personal, so I kept my mouth firmly shut.

Adrian paused for a few seconds to think of another boring question.

'So, do you have a favourite colour then?' He asked.

And I replied, 'Dark energy does not have a colour, but without it, the universe could not exist.'

I think I may have strayed off-topic with this answer, but I wasn't about to tell Adrian Wilkes why my special wiring sometimes makes me say the first thing that comes to mind. Thankfully, he didn't ask any more stupid questions.

Finally, after what felt like the longest walk in history, we arrived at his mum's place above *East Winslow Plumbing Supplies* at the far end of the High Street. We climbed three flights of concrete steps and stopped at a green door. Next to it, a sign said:

'BEWARE OF THE DOG!'

The picture was of a hound so terrifying it made Trevor look like a fluffy little chick. I was about to turn and run when Adrian laughed and said, 'Don't worry about the sign. It's only there to scare people away; we don't *actually* have a dog!'

He reached into his backpack and pulled out a brass key that had somehow found its way inside a half-eaten cucumber sandwich. Probably a leftover from lunchtime. He scraped away the mayonnaise and was about to insert the slimy key in the lock when the door opened. It was Mrs Wilkes with a great big sunny smile and short blond hair. She wore a pink tee-shirt with the words *Life Is Not A Rehearsal* embossed in silver sequins on the front.

'Hi Mum,' Adrian said, pushing passed into the narrow hallway.

Mrs Wilkes rolled her eyes and shook her head.

'So... you must be Timothy? Or would you rather I called you Timmy? I've heard so much about you from Adrian. He says you two are best friends.'

'BEST FRIENDS?!' Wow, I thought, that was news to me!

I was so confused by all the questions that I didn't know what to reply to first, so I decided not to say anything at all. Not, at least, until I had time to consider what it would be like to be called *Timmy* by someone other than Mum.

Mrs Wilkes closed the front door and I followed

her into the kitchen. Adrian was already plunging a huge slice of pizza, intended for tea time, into his mouth. Sticky tomato sauce skids coloured the sides of his mouth where he'd quickly forced it in. This was a pretty pathetic attempt to conceal his greed. Still, I didn't dwell on his massive personality flaws for long, because the table was filled with tons of stuff I really like. There were chocolate mini muffins (from the bakery in the High Street), tins of fizzy orange juice (unsweetened), sandwiches (white bread with the crusts cut away), peanut butter (the smooth type), and marmalade (without the nasty hard bits). It was almost like being at home; as though someone had told Mrs Wilkes *exactly* what food to buy. I even began to think that this 'having friends' thing may not be such a bad idea after all.

'So... have you decided what you'd like me to call you yet?' Mrs Wilkes asked again.

Only then, did it occur to me that if I let her call me *Timmy,* Adrian would also start calling me *Timmy.* Then Mr Willowby would, as would Cynthia in Student Services, and then Clare Feathersdale and Amanda Goldbloom would catch on, and everyone at Highcrest, and the staff at AstroWorld. Then it would go viral across the internet. Within days, everyone on the planet with access to WIFI would think my name was 'Timmy,' the nickname I hate because it sounds a bit like 'Billy'—the disgusting kid who called me a weirdo when I was seven.

'Well, I suppose you can call me *Timothy*.' I said, realising there were no other reasonable options.

'Excellent, that's settled then, Timothy it is! You can call me *Sue* if you like.'

So, there I was at the kitchen table with Sue Wilkes sitting to my right and Adrian opposite. I'm not sure how long I didn't speak for, but it felt like ages and it was all getting pretty uncomfortable.

Adrian hadn't said anything either. He was far too busy stuffing pizza and chocolate mini muffins into his mouth—practically at the same time. It wasn't until Mrs Wilkes mentioned the unusually large full moon flooding the kitchen with light the previous evening that I felt the urge to turn my thoughts into words. Lots and lots of words.

I knew she was doing that embarrassing small talk thing that grown-ups do to get the conversation going, but it didn't stop me from pointing out that her assertions about the moon being unusually large were totally incorrect.

'The moon *hadn't* suddenly grown in size. ONLY AN IDIOT WOULD THINK THAT! It was, quite obviously, an optical illusion. Anyone who knows the first thing about science would know the moon looked bigger than usual because of the atmospheric conditions in combination with an atypical orbital trajectory. SURELY ANYONE WITH HALF A BRAIN CELL WOULD KNOW *THAT!*' I said, using my best irritated voice.

Mrs Wilkes stopped smiling and did that scrunched-up eyebrow thing for a few seconds, and said: 'Well... you obviously know a lot more about astronomy than I do. How long has it been an interest of yours?'

And the really strange thing is, I didn't know the answer. Weirder still, I couldn't even remember how I'd become so obsessed with the subject in the first place. Much like when I was seven and all I could think about were bearded dragon lizards. Then, when I was eight, all I wanted to think about was the colour blue. Everything had to be blue. My bedroom walls, my clothes, my shoes, my underwear, my hot choco-late mug. It didn't matter which shade of blue, as long as it was blue: sky blue, navy blue, Chelsea blue, aqua blue. The funny thing is I don't even like blue that much anymore. Don't get me wrong, as a colour it's pretty decent. Definitely better than putrid pink. But I'm much keener on green these days. It reminds me of serene views across the Yorkshire Dales and the cabbage Mum makes for Sunday lunch. Ahhh— Sunday lunch... I can almost taste it. Crispy golden potatoes soaked in gravy, soft white chicken, carrots, and chestnut stuffing...

Mrs Wilkes cleared her throat again, much louder this time.

'Anyway,' she said, changing the subject. 'Has Adrian told you about his new binoculars? He drove me around-the-bend for a set after he watched a TV program about an undercover surveillance detective. They're not cheap ones either. I've only just finished paying off for them. Perhaps you and him could team up and become stargazers. You could bring your telescope over after school and the two of you could look for UFOs and signs of alien life—how exciting!'

I couldn't tell if Mrs Wilkes was joking or not, but once again, I felt compelled to set her straight.

'UFOS DO NOT EXIST! There's not a single shred of evidence to support any of the reported sightings. People say they've seen strange lights in the sky and they turn out to be Chinese lanterns or expertly faked pictures. Sometimes people are fooled by sunlight reflecting off an aeroplane. And sometimes the lights are from a car at night on a road cut high into the side of a hill and—'

'OKAY TIMOTHY, I GET THE IDEA! I'm sorry. I was only joking about UFOs. I just thought it would be fun for you and Adrian to meet up occasionally after school...'

Adrian wiped away a chocolate-muffin-face-skid with the back of his hand and said: 'But I hate astronomy! I thought we were going to play football in the garden or something, like when Jamie comes over. We watch funny videos on the computer and play games. But this isn't fun, it's boring. Timothy is boring, and I don't even know why you told me to invite him over in the first place!'

'ADRIAN! STOP IT! THAT'S ENOUGH!'

Mrs Wilkes glared at him as though he'd been caught, red-handed, revealing state secrets to the enemy.

Luckily for Adrian, The National Anthem suddenly blasted out through his mum's diamond-encrusted phone. The melody was played on something that sounded like rapidly deflating bagpipes. She caught the vibrating phone just as it was about to topple from the microwave and onto the floor. Adrian sighed with relief, and so did I when she swiped and killed the music. That call must have saved him from getting into some pretty serious trouble.

Mrs Wilkes held the phone in place with her shoulder and began clearing the table.

'Hi, Barbara... yes, he's fine. Okay, so you'll collect him soon? Great, I'll let him know.'

Seven minutes and eleven seconds later, the doorbell rang. It was Mum.

'Thanks for everything, Sue, I'll call you tonight.' Her voice trailed off into silence, as though the end of the sentence was being transmitted secretly, by thought and a knowing smile. Somehow, Mrs Wilkes knew what Mum meant. She nodded and said, 'Okay, no problem. Let's speak later.'

'GOODBYE, TIMOTHY. IT WAS LOVELY HAVING YOU OVER!' Mrs Wilkes shouted from the top of the stairs as we climbed into our car and slammed the doors shut.

A few minutes later (I can't be any more precise than this because I was too tired to count) we pulled into our driveway, and Mum switched the engine off.

We sat in silence for a while, staring out through the windscreen. The sky was black, and rows of street lamps radiated like orange glow worms on grey concrete sticks into the distance.

'So, how did it go then—at Adrian's?' Mum finally asked.

'Well, it could have been worse, I suppose. But I wouldn't exactly say it was fun. Mrs Wilkes is quite nice, but she doesn't know much about astronomy so we could never be friends.'

I think Mum was just about to ask a follow-up question when the light came on in our house. The warm-yellow spread halfway across the lawn and almost up to the roof. Higher up, the chimney was still a dark silhouette against a wash of faded stars. Through the car window, I watched Dad walk across the living room and drop down into an armchair. I could almost hear the sound of a newspaper rustling through his fingers and a boiled kettle pouring an evening brew. Upstairs, Schrodinger would be resting on a bed of seaweed by now; ready for a chat before bedtime. It all seemed so cosy and safe. But then I began to wonder what Adrian might be doing: probably busy on his phone, sending *not* funny jokes about me to his '*not boring*' friends. And this is exactly why I hate the idea of getting to know people—it's all too complicated.

I don't need friends. I already have everything I need for a happy life. And it's all right here, right now, at 47 Eaton Drive.

21 THE MORNING AFTER

The morning after my, *could have been a lot worse,* visit to Adrian's house

I FELT EXHAUSTED EVEN though I'd been asleep for hours. I couldn't stop thinking about Adrian. If I'd thought about it at the time, I would have got angry and asked why he'd said, '*I don't even know why you told me to invite him*—meaning me—*over in the first place!*' But, as usual, I didn't think about it properly till hours later when I was alone in my room. That's when I lay on my bed and think about all the things I wished I'd said that day and all the things I wished I hadn't.

I must admit, though, I was beginning to feel

pretty angry about Adrian calling me boring. If you ask me, HE'S the one that's boring. The only questions HE could think of asking on the way over to his place were about football, food and colours—UNINTERESTING OR *WHAT?!*

I spoke to Mum about what Adrian had said, and apparently, the reason Sue Wilkes told him to invite me over was because she's a special-needs teaching assistant at St John's over in South Dunsford. And that she was used to supporting children like me—whatever *that* meant. Mum and her thought it would be a chance for me to have some 'making-friends' practice with Adrian. Well, I wish they'd asked me first. If they had, I would definitely have said, 'FORGET IT!'

Well—so much for democracy. I guess *that* only applies to grown-ups.

Anyway, Mum said that after I'd gone to bed, Sue Wilkes called and told her that for a first attempt at 'making-friends,' things had gone quite well. She also said that I was extremely clever and had excellent table manners (not like her 'ape of a son —Adrian!')

Well, *that's* stating the obvious—obviously! But then they agreed that Adrian should come along on our next trip to AstroWorld so that I could improve my making-friends skills even further.

'BUT THAT'S THE WORST IDEA, *EVER!*' I shouted at Mum.

Just the thought of it made my belly rumble and my thoughts explode. I mean... me, plus Adrian Wilkes, plus AstroWorld! That must be the most ridiculous equation of all time. Einstein would turn in his grave if he heard it—not literally, of course, that would be impossible. And not only *that*: why was everyone telling me that I've got to learn how to make friends? I must have told Mum a thousand times how I like things just the way they are. But as usual, no one listens to *my* opinion around here.

Then I tried to convince Mum that Adrian hated *anything* that involved using that grey squashy thing trapped inside his hideous skull—otherwise known as a brain. And that he would absolutely hate Astro-World. But she wasn't buying any of it and insisted that being with other people is good for one's emotional wellbeing. She backed up her point by saying how the doctor who tested me for the 'A-word' said I needed to 'Challenge my fears,' and 'Broaden my horizons.'

I reminded Mum that I already *was* broadening

my horizons—thank you very much! 'Because the universe is, contrary to the laws of conventional physics, expanding faster all the time when it should, in fact, be slowing down. So, as a consequence, my horizons were *also* expanding faster than they should be—just not in a way that means I need to have friends.'

Mum squeezed her eyebrows together and nodded slowly up and down. This may have meant she didn't quite get my analogy, and if I'm being totally honest, I'm not sure I did either.

But I wasn't finished... 'And not only *that*, did you know there's a thing in Switzerland called *The Large Hadron Collider*? Scientists use it to smash particles into each other at almost the speed of light?'

Mum said that now I was definitely straying from the topic. And, in any case, although what I'd said about Switzerland sounded like a question, it was more of a statement that didn't require an answer. Then she told me to eat my breakfast and get ready for school. She turned towards the sink and squirted green washing-up liquid on the breakfast plates. I think she may have been angry with me for being different to the type of child she'd hoped for. I could sense angry energy waves swirling around the back of her head. But then—I suppose they could just as easily have been *sad* energy waves. Sad because she's so upset about all the 'A-word' stuff and how it makes me get things wrong all the time. Sad because Dad's always saying, 'FOR GOD'S SAKE, TIMOTHY! CAN'T YOU JUST GIVE A SIMPLE ANSWER TO A SIMPLE QUESTION?' Sad because, for the rest of my time on Earth, she knows people will say, *Timothy Blossom, the boy from East Winslow whose special wiring makes him so totally and officially different.*

22 ELEPHANTS AND PURPLE HAIR

ACCORDING to Cynthia in Student Services, I had a stonking great elephant in the middle of my room. How it got there was a mystery. But she said it would not leave until I began to talk about stuff I was worried about.

'What stuff?' I asked. 'About elephants? I need to talk about elephants, and they'll disappear?'

'Yes, if you want to put it like that,' Cynthia replied —at least I *think* it was Cynthia. Her voice certainly sounded familiar. But something was different, and to be quite honest it was all getting a little weird. I thought I was supposed to be talking about my feelings, but instead, the person posing as Cynthia kept going on about large grey mammals with trunks!

It was a Friday afternoon and we were having one of our fortnightly chats. Cynthia will usually say something like, 'So—how are things going then,' and I'll say, 'Fine thanks,' because I'm polite. And also because figuring out what people *really* mean is too much like hard work. It's much easier to just say, 'I'm fine, thanks,' instead.

But on this particular visit to Student Services, it was clear that something *big* had changed, and it was all I could think about.

Miraculously, the sculptured tower that had been Cynthia's hair the previous day was now a purple flow of curls reaching to her waist. And those brilliant astrological signs embossed in silver on sky-blue fingernails, were now a wash of violet swirls graduating to a rainbow palette of pastel pink. I kept glancing at the holiday snaps on Cynthia's desk, and then at her to see if I could spot any similarities in bone structure and skin tone, but because I'm so rubbish at recognising people's faces—mainly because I never really look at anyone straight on—I still couldn't say for sure if this was the *real* Cynthia.

The seconds on the big white wall clock were ticking by louder than ever, and the person who said she was Cynthia was still looking at me as if it was my turn to speak. But all I could think about were elephants and purple hair.

'Never mind—let's talk about something else,' the woman who *may* have been Cynthia said in her best, kind voice.

'Did you know that there are lots of famous people with aut—'

I quickly stuck my fingers in my ears and closed my eyes.

'I HATE THAT WORD. AND I HATE THE OTHER WORD THAT ENDS IN *ISTIC* EVEN MORE. THAT'S WHY I CALL IT THE *"A-WORD." I THOUGHT YOU KNEW THAT!*' I screamed.

She told me to take some deep breaths and then apologised for upsetting me. She said that when I get home after school I should type into my computer: *famous people with AUT—*. And that I wouldn't need to type '*ISM*' on the end, as all the good stuff would automatically appear in the search results without it. She said I'd be pleasantly surprised by the results— and she wasn't wrong. The woman, who I was now seventy per cent sure *was* the real Cynthia, had definitely earned her place on my new *circle of trust* list. When I got home, I even promoted her above Dad who'd been kind of grumpy that morning. I added her name in shades of violet, purple and pink to match her new hair and nails. And as a special *thank you* for providing me with such an intriguingly brilliant new search term.

Later That Evening

After dinner, I switched on my computer, and as usual, waited impatiently for it to boot-up.

'One day,' I said to Schrodinger, 'computers will be controlled by thought alone. They will respond immediately to our every telepathic command. Until then we are at the mercy of all those ones and zeros passing through a network of archaic components at the speed of a slow worm—TOTALLY ridiculous!'

I'm pretty sure Schrodinger would have agreed, if he hadn't been snoozing in the gravel. There he was, snoring silently away in gulps of cloudy green water. He's always preferred the simple life—the quiet life. I can *definitely* relate to that!

Anyway, I brought my thoughts back to the task at hand and logged in using the password I cannot reveal.

Finally, I was able to click and connect to the World Wide Web. To enter its vast portal of knowledge. To browse its many halls of learning without leaving the safety of my bedroom. I paused briefly; hands poised over the keyboard, and began to type: *Famous people with aut—*

35,900,000 results were found in 0.78 seconds—SERIOUSLY impressive!

There were lists upon lists of famous people who were thought to have the 'A-word.' I could have scrolled for a thousand years without reaching the end. There were actors, artists, musicians, authors, mathematicians, models, TV presenters, basketball players, golfers, politicians, doctors, inventors and billionaire social media company owners. And then I saw it. A name I could not, in a gazillion light-years, have expected to see on a list of famous people with the 'A-word': ALBERT EINSTEIN (born, Germany 1875. Died, Princeton Medical Center, USA 1955).

Well—I nearly fell off my chair. There he was in glorious black and white. Crazy hair and wild eyes staring back at me through my computer screen. The man who'd said: *'Energy equals mass times the speed of light squared.'*

So, I *wasn't* the only person in the world with the 'A-word' after all. Cynthia was right. I really *was* special like they say on those boring diversity days. I mean, who else around here could boast they shared genetic characteristics with the greatest scientist of all time? The man who *also* probably had the 'A-word?' My hero, the totally brilliant, the one and only, ALBERT EINSTEIN!

23 BLAST-OFF!

IT WAS SUNDAY, October 17th, the day I'd hoped would never come. The day Adrian was coming over so I could have some more making-friends practice. The plan was that he'd get here around noon, in time for lunch, and afterwards, Dad would take the two of us to AstroWorld.

I hadn't slept much the previous night. Every time I tried, Adrian's face was two inches from mine; his hot breath coating my skin in human-goat-slime. It was horrible. Then I'd suddenly snap into being awake again. I'd watch the green numbers on my bedside clock tick by, then drift away once more for an hour or two.

At breakfast, I could barely keep my eyes open. I

tried hard not to be in a bad mood, but couldn't help it and said some pretty bad things to Mum that I wished I hadn't. At one point I screamed at her louder than I ever had before.

'I HATE ADRIAN. WHY DID YOU INVITE HIM OVER? I HATE PEOPLE, AND I HATE YOU!'

I threw my toast at the wall and ran upstairs. I hid in the corner of my room next to Schrodinger's tank and tried to cry to let the pressure out of my brain. A few minutes later I heard the door squeak open. Schrodinger dived behind the pink shell we'd found on a beach in Cornwall, and I covered my face with my hands because I didn't want anyone to see me.

'How are you feeling, Timmy?'

Mum's soft voice drifted over me like a warm fluffy cloud. I thought she was going to be angry with me for shouting, but she wasn't, and I began to feel a bit calmer.

'Look... I know you're worried about Adrian coming over today, but I promise, nothing bad is going to happen.'

'But what happens if neither of us can think of anything good to talk about? That would be the worst, most embarrassing thing ever.'

'But the more practice you get talking to people

your own age, the easier it will get. Try asking him about his hobbies. Ask him if he has any pets, and how long he's lived in East Winslow. It's called *small talk*, and anyone who achieves anything in life is skilled in the art of small talk. It's something most people can learn to do if they try hard enough. Just remember this: the worst thing that can ever possibly happen is never usually that bad. Be brave, be strong, and think big.'

'Wow, Mum, that was really deep!' I was about to say, when, from behind the hands that still shielded my face, I heard the floorboards creak gently under the weight of her slippered footsteps. My squeaky bedroom door that Dad says he'll fix, but never does, clicked closed.

Two Hours, Four Minutes and Fifty-Two Seconds Later...

I was busy in my room typing things like, *how to do small talk and achieve big things in life*, into the internet.

0.58 seconds and 250,000,000 results later, all I could find were videos of loud people standing in front of posh cars yelling about how *anyone* could become a millionaire in six weeks. All I had to do was sign up for their free, five-step-plan, then sit back and watch the cash roll in. WOW! This was definitely something I should mention to Dad. He's always complaining that he doesn't have enough money.

Suddenly, there was a loud triple-knock on my door. It was an unfamiliar knock that couldn't have been made by Mum or Dad. They know the rule about only knocking in *even* numbers. An unusually large splash whipped from Schrodinger's orange tail and landed with a splat next to me on the carpet. Back and forth he raced across the surface before diving into the seaweed. I panicked and turned my computer off from the wall switch without shutting down properly first. This was a rule I'd never broken before and knew there'd be some pretty terrible consequences as a result. And I wasn't wrong.

For a large, magnified second, other than my thumping heartbeat, all was quiet and still. But then came the dreaded, never-heard-in-this-house-before voice of Adrian Wilkes. He was in MY house, outside MY bedroom, invading MY space, and about to infect MY air. I wanted to hide under the bed, but instead raced towards the door and squeezed it open just wide enough to see out. And there he was, the most annoying person in the world, holding a box of chocolate mini muffins and a bottle of fizzy orange (unsweetened).

'Well, are you going to invite me in then, or what? These muffins are getting heavy—I can feel my arms dropping off.'

But surely, I wondered, those mini muffins could not be heavy enough to pull a boy's arms from their sockets? Or maybe they were...?

'How heavy are they then, exactly?' I asked.

'How heavy is *what*?' He said, making one of those confused faces he pulls in class when Mr Willowby asks him a question about science.

'The chocolate mini muffins, of course,' I replied. 'How heavy are they?'

'How am I supposed to know?! All I know is I'm getting really bored out here. When are you going to let me in?'

Luckily, before I had to use the brilliant excuse I'd been practising for days as to why he couldn't possibly, not in at least a million years, *EVER*, enter my room, Mum's voice bellowed up from the kitchen:

'FOOD'S READY, BOYS. COME AND GET IT!'

Well—I'd never seen Adrian move so fast! He was like an elephant slug on square wheels, thumping down the staircase in three clumsy bounces. I waited for the chandelier to stop swinging from the vibration and began my descent two steps at a time.

To say that lunch was tense was an understatement bigger than Saturn and all of its rings. For a start, I hate eating in front of people I'm not used to. I get really self-conscious and worry about being stared at. This is the main reason I sit alone in the school canteen, facing the wall. Plus, I wouldn't want anyone making small talk as a sneaky ruse to share my sandwiches.

Adrian, oblivious as ever, didn't seem to care about who saw him eat. There he was, tucking into the roast lamb before I'd even had a chance to sit down. It was like he hadn't seen food for days. Gravy was everywhere: splattered on the tablecloth and smeared across his face all the way up to a floppy fringe. The brown slime was all over his hands from pulling away the fat with his fingers and was probably even on his shoes—although I didn't bother to check. And when Mum asked him if he'd like some more, he belched and held out his plate so that Mum could load it up again. Then it was head down once more, deep into the steaming food without coming up for air even once. He was a mess before we'd even started on dessert.

Amongst those in the know, Mum's homemade apple pie and custard is regarded as something of a speciality. Each chunk of apple is carefully sliced, diced, tested for consistency then soaked in lemon juice overnight. The following morning, it's baked at a temperature of one hundred and eighty degrees in a fan-assisted oven, then coated in a secret cinnamon-based topping. This is a recipe passed down through generations of proud Blossoms dating all the way back to William the Conqueror—or so the story goes.

Not that Adrian cared. Before I'd even placed a napkin to protect my shirt from custard spills, he'd dived in; shovelling heaped spoonfuls into his mouth faster than he could swallow. Yellow juice dripped from his chin and unchewed apple puffed out his cheeks fatter than a squirrel hoarding nuts for winter. It was totally disgusting, and at one point I even had to close my eyes to avoid throwing up!

Finally, resting in the aftermath of the epic battle, Adrian slumped back in his chair, bloated and exhausted. He took a mighty gulp of air and wiped a dribble of custard sweat from his brow.

'I'm stuffed!' He said, suppressing another belch under his breath. 'I think I need a lie-down.'

'No time for that, Son!' Dad said—looking up at the wall clock ticking steadily towards *launch-time*. 'We've got a train to catch.'

AstroWorld is just a short walk from West Cranford station. Normally, if I'm in a good mood, the moment Dad spots the illuminated plastic Earth globe spinning slowly over the main entrance, he'll shout, '1... 2... 3 BLAST-OFF!' And I'll sprint faster than I ever can on school sports day through the glass swing-doors. But, today, probably due to the stress of Adrian being there, when Dad shouted, '1... 2... 3 BLAST-OFF!' I looked down at the ground, and then half at Adrian instead.

I must admit, I felt a bit embarrassed about all the pretend *blast-off* stuff. But Adrian wasn't in the slightest bit embarrassed. Still fully loaded from lunch, he leapt into the air and made a brilliant roaring sound with his mouth. It was just like Apollo 12 lifting off from Cape Canaveral in 1969. At warp speed, Adrian tore across the car park, leaving Astro-

World's entrance doors swinging off their hinges in a whirl of galactic dust.

'WOW! THAT WAS AMAZING!' My eyes bulged wide from the excitement of Adrian's extraordinary blast-off. I could contain myself no longer. 'I... 2... 3!' I screamed and launched into his identical flight path through the still swinging doors. And as for Dad, well he was left way behind in the car park, like a slow-moving mothership.

It was the beginning of December, and AstroWorld's display cabinets were dressed in silver and gold tinsel; ready for the best season of all: Christmas.

'Incredible!' I heard myself say. It was like all of my non-scary dreams had come true at once. I honestly didn't know where to look first. Towering rocket-shaped Christmas trees pointed skywards through pine-scented air. And presents draped in shiny baubles shouted, 'BUY ME, BUY ME!' In words only I could hear. At least a million fairy lights twinkled in time to, *'Have Yourself a Merry Little Christmas'*—the original 1944 version by Judy Garland. My favourite version of my favourite ever yuletide song.

Adrian, who'd suddenly landed next to me after several AstroWorld orbits and was almost able to breathe again without squeaking through his lungs, reached over and placed his hand on my shoulder. 'OMG!' He gasped, accidentally burying his right leg in a polystyrene snowdrift. 'This place is amazing! Now I understand why you're *so* obsessed with astronomy.'

Together, Adrian and I ventured forward along the aisles, deeper and deeper into Christmas: beyond time and space, like galactic explorers, until the translucent skylights became dark with night and splattered by an autumn shower.

'OKAY BOYS, CHOOSE SOMETHING QUICKLY. IT'S GETTING LATE AND WE'VE GOT A TRAIN TO CATCH!'

Dad's voice crashed through planet Christmas like a heatwave in Lapland. In an instant, Adrian and I were back down to Earth with a mighty, unfestive bump.

I took the handful of change left over from my birthday money, out of my pocket, and gave it, along with a rolled-up poster of Einstein to the unfriendly lady behind the cash till. She had on a red Santa hat with gold trim.

'That will be £3.99,' she said, without smiling once or saying please. 'Would you like a carrier bag? If you do, it's another ten pence.'

I couldn't work out if I had enough money, so I said, 'No thanks,' and stood to one side as Adrian approached. He'd bought a bag of astronaut-shaped jelly babies and had eaten the lot whilst waiting in the queue. He handed the empty polythene bag to the cashier who scanned the bar code.

'That will be £1.75. Would you like a carrier bag? If you do, it's another ten pence.'

My telepathy skills are pretty good these days, and I could tell Adrian wasn't happy about paying all that money for a bag of air with a residue of sugar at the bottom—even though *he* was the one who'd emptied it!

'No—I do *not* want a carrier bag, thank you very much!' He replied, snatching his purchase from the unChristmasy cashier's grasp.

'NEXT!' She shouted at Dad.

Although he looked like he was queueing, he was only there in a supervisory role. He never buys anything for himself at AstroWorld. I guess astronomy's not really his thing.

The light had gone by the time we boarded the train home. We watched the dark outlines of trees and buildings rush by to the rhythm of steel wheels on bumpy tracks. Nobody spoke at first; we didn't need to. Words could not express how unexpectedly brilliant the afternoon had been. Adrian even gave me his last astronaut-shaped jelly baby. It looked like a squashed purple Neil Armstrong. It had been hiding in sugar at the bottom of the bag the whole time— revealing itself only when the train jerked to a sudden halt at Wades Cross. And because Neil Armstrong had taken such a gigantic leap for mankind, I made sure it lasted all the way home.

'Your next stop will be East Winslow, please do not leave your luggage unattended'—the posh recorded lady announced over the carriage sound system.

'AstroWorld, AstroWorld, the store with a universe of galactic Christmas gifts!' Adrian and I sang over, and over, and over again to the tune of Jingle Bells. It wasn't an easy fit, but together, somehow, we made it work.

24 THE CHRISTMAS PARTY

THERE WAS something cold in the air, and the cold thing was called December 20th. It was the final day of school before the holidays, and the day of High-crest Manor's Christmas party.

Christmas was the only time of year that made me wonder if magic, in the shape of Santa, might actually exist. Of course, I wouldn't admit this to anyone, especially not to Mr Willowby. I wouldn't want him to think I'd lost my braininess and had turned my back on science. And anyway, even if Santa *was* real, he'd definitely need some new tactics to keep up with all the latest trends in DIY. Most people brick their fireplaces up these days and replace them with wood burners or gas fires. Mum turned *our* fireplace into a trendy white space filled with scented candles, crystals and dried flowers. There's just no way Santa could chisel his way through all the blocked-up chimneys and still deliver gifts to every child in the world before dawn on Christmas morning. Impossible.

Anyway, this year, the school Christmas party began with a short firework display and a pretty boring speech from 'Santa' about world peace. He went on, and on, and on about how we must love our fellow humans. YUK! For a moment, I thought I'd have to hold hands with whoever was standing next to me, and hug, and sing *We are the World!* Thankfully, it never came to that. I think I can speak for every kid there when I say how relieved I was when Santa bellowed a final, 'HO HO HO,' then disappeared back inside his grotto to organise the presents.

Practically everyone who had anything to do with Highcrest Manor was at the party: Adrian, and all the other kids in my class (whose names I'd *still* not bothered to learn), Mr Willowby, Cynthia from Student Services, Ellen Ford the headteacher, everyone's mums, dads, brothers and sisters. Even someone's grandpa showed up for some free, festive grub and a glass of Christmas cheer. There were hot mince pies, turkey sandwiches, fruit cakes decorated with icing that looked like snow, gallons of fizzy orange and cola, steaming jugs of mulled wine spiced with cinnamon and ginger for the parents, and silver bowls of water for the reindeer—yeah, sure! Hogged instead by a tiny, pampered pooch dressed in a colourful *Merry Christmas* jacket.

The sports hall was a sight to behold, unrecognisable, in fact. Thankfully, without the usual disgusting smell of sweaty trainers. The place was decked out with plastic pine trees and every other type of festive decoration imaginable. Disco lights danced in big colourful circles, and Christmas carols blared louder than my thoughts.

Clare and Amanda, inseparable as ever, seemed to be enjoying themselves. They wore identical woolly jumpers emblazoned with elves and flying reindeer. They were holding hands, as usual, singing along to the disco version of *Frosty the Snowman*. Amanda knew most of the words and almost sang in tune, but Clare was only miming—*really* badly—her mouth wasn't even close to making the right shapes. Amanda kept laughing and pointing at her every time she went wrong. Then they tried to synchronise their dance routines. Well, if you ask me, I think they should stick to what they're good at—getting good marks for homework!

Mum spent most of the party talking to Sue Wilkes, and I spent most of it hiding behind her. They must have drunk at least four glasses of mulled wine each; possibly even five, and their empty throw-away cups became a big heap of recycling on the serving counter.

'DON'T YOU KNOW THE PLANET IS IN CRISIS?! DROWNING IN A SEA OF PLASTIC?!' I felt like saying. But because Mum looked so happy, I didn't want to start lecturing her on how she was destroying the ozone layer and poisoning the oceans.

Now, it could have been a reflection from the flashing disco lights, but after a few drinks, Mum's cheeks began to glow like red Christmas baubles. She kept fanning her face with her hand and giggling—as was Sue Wilkes. They were laughing and linking arms, just like Clare and Amanda always do. I hadn't seen Mum so relaxed in ages, what with all the 'A-word' stuff and Dad going on all the time about 'getting the chop' from his job. Seeing Mum like this made me feel a bit less sad than I usually get at school parties. Although, she wasn't quite as happy the next day when she woke up with, *'The headache from hell,'* and had to go back to bed for a few hours after breakfast. My guess was that she'd probably caught the headache from Sue Wilkes, who'd also looked a bit wobbly on the way home.

One thing I've never really understood about parties is why people think they're such a great idea in the first place. All of that noise, and joking around, and having to make embarrassing small talk with people you'd rather ignore. What a nightmare! But the main reason I hate parties is that I don't know what I'm supposed to do when I'm at them. And at *this*, my very first 'A-word' party, it feels like everyone's looking at me. Laughing and pointing and saying:

'Look, there's Timothy Blossom, the officially different kid from Mr Willowby's class.'

At least, that's what I imagine everyone's saying.

I must admit though, I didn't feel quite as self-conscious as I normally do at these things. I suppose my newfound confidence might have something to do with the fact I'm now thirteen years, two months and fourteen days old. Or perhaps it's got something to do with that unexpectedly brilliant afternoon at Astro-World with Adrian. I hadn't realised he was so interested in astronomy. *That* was a secret he'd kept well-hidden for two years.

Anyway, getting back to the Christmas party. It was just before the end, and all the non-wobbly parents were helping the school staff tidy up. They were rushing around with brooms and filling black bin liners with half-eaten food. *Silent Night* had just finished playing for the third time in a row, and Mr Willowby was now, for some inexplicable reason, wearing headphones and controlling the music. He kept making stupid announcements over the microphone in an American (or possibly Australian) accent. I suppose it was mildly amusing the first few times he shouted, *'DJ WILLOWS IS IN THE HOUSE!'* But after thirty-two times, it became so cringingly embarrassing that I had to stick my fingers in my ears. And then, to make matters even worse, he started doing the *Moonwalk* and some weird robot moves he'd learnt in 1982. That's when I closed my eyes and tried to bury my face in Mum's handbag. It was all pretty sad. If you ask me, old people like him (I think he's forty-three) should definitely *not* be allowed to control the music at parties—or dance in public, for that matter.

I was just recovering from all the embarrassment

when I heard mum say, 'Hello Clare—Amanda. Gosh, look how big you are. I remember when you were both in nappies! How wonderful it is that you're still best friends after all these years.'

Clare and Amanda looked at each other and giggled.

'Fancy another drink before home-time, girls?' Mum asked, filling their cups with cola that didn't have any fizz left because someone had left the top off the bottle. They gulped it down, and just as they were about to head off for a final dance, Mum said the worst thing she'd said in her entire life. She looked at me and said, 'Go on, Timmy, why don't you go and dance with Clare and Amanda while I finish talking to Sue.'

Well... I could feel my face contort into strange angry shapes. My eyes squinted in half-closed rage squeezing hate in Mum's direction.

'I DON'T WANT TO DANCE. I NEVER DANCE. I HATE PEOPLE WHO DANCE. AND I HATE *YOU!*' Came a deep, gravel-toned-devil-voice I'd not heard exit my mouth before.

'Come on, Timmy,' Mum said, undeterred and smiling. 'Lighten up, it's Christmas!'

She winked at Clare, who giggled again. Then

Amanda, who was a lot stronger than I could have imagined, grabbed my hand and pulled me right into the middle of the dance floor. Immediately, everyone formed a tight circle around us and began to clap their hands in time to the music. I could not escape. Amanda was jiggling my arms up and down and back and forth, whilst Clare made loud whooping noises; bouncing from one foot to the other. The disco lights flashed brighter with each burst of red, blue and green, as Amanda twirled me around and around in a dizzying shamanic trance.

Suddenly, someone lurched violently forward through the crowd and landed heavily on my left foot. 'OUCH!' I screamed, but I could not be heard above the music. It was clumsy Adrian Wilkes, thrusting his hideous body into the middle of our crazy circle. He was like a two-ton ballerina wrestling an invisible gorilla. I'd never seen anything like it. And judging by the expression on everyone's faces, neither had they.

'TOO MUCH SUGAR!' Amanda shouted; laughing and pointing at Adrian who'd turned into a sort of human Catherine wheel. Faster and faster he span; his arms punching the air like hopelessly out of time fleshy pistons to a beat only *he* could hear. His eyes were closed, and a brown fringe, stuck by sweat and snot, clung to the side of his freckled nose. Adrian was a whirling haze of uncontrolled motion, without rhyme or reason, poise or purpose. As if possessed by an alien life-force, desperate to escape his body before the song ended.

Suddenly, Adrian lost his balance. His legs had moved too fast for his body. He collapsed sideways onto Amanda, who fell on top of Clare, who tried to save herself by grabbing hold of my shirt sleeve. The next thing I knew, all four of us were laying in a heap on the floor, laughing hysterically until we could barely breathe. This had never happened to me before, and I felt so free, so alive. I couldn't believe that I was *joining in.* That I was actually laughing with other people. Then I saw that Mum was also laughing. So was Sue Wilkes, and Mr Willowby, and Cynthia from Student Services, and headteacher Ellen Ford. Then all the other kids from my class began rolling around on the floor in fits of laughter. Even the DJ, who'd thankfully regained control of the record decks from Mr Willowby, had tears streaming from his eyes and was forced to stop the music. Santa couldn't carry on either and dropped his sack. He was, 'HO HO HO-ING,' so loud, his face turned the same colour as his outfit. The grotto line was backed up longer than a black Friday sale at AstroWorld. But the *queuers* didn't care—they were howling with laughter as well.

After about ten minutes of unexpected mayhem, the boring overhead lights came on in the sports hall and overpowered the disco lights. It was like someone sensible had suddenly decided to turn the fun off. Slowly, everyone made their way towards the exit sign and out into the cold December night.

Amanda and Clare, who were still giggling, along with a few other kids who seemed to know who I was, called out, 'Goodnight Timothy Blossom, have a great Christmas, see you next year!' I nodded in their direction and very nearly replied, 'Thanks—you too.' But I'm not ready for that type of conversation yet, so I waved at them and had nice thoughts instead.

Then, just when I thought things couldn't get any more Christmas-ier, Mum said: 'OH WOW, TIMOTHY—LOOK!'

Whilst we'd been at the party, the sky had opened and painted the streets and houses thick with clean white snow. Heavy lumps were still falling fast like cold confetti from Santa's sleigh. It was perfect. Just how Christmas was supposed to look. It didn't even seem to matter anymore that those 'A-word' tests had confirmed that I was now officially different. Because at that precise moment, and for the first time ever, I Timothy James Arthur Blossom: age thirteen years, two months and fourteen days, also felt officially brilliant.

AFTERWORD

If you enjoyed reading Timothy Blossom – Officially Brilliant, please consider leaving a review.

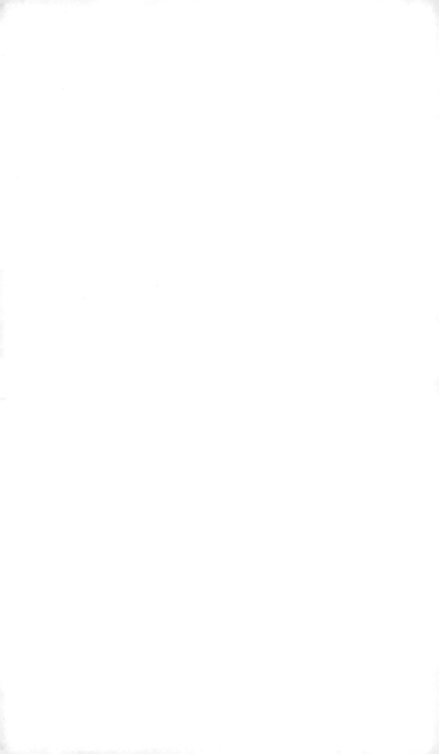

Printed in Great Britain
by Amazon